Two
Hugs for
Survival

Two Hugs for Survival

Strategies for Effective Parenting

Dr. Harold A. Minden

McClelland and Stewart

McClelland and Stewart Limited
The Canadian Publishers
25 Hollinger Road
Toronto, Ontario
M4B 3G2

Canadian Cataloguing in Publication Data

Minden, Harold A. (Harold Allen)
  Two hugs for survival

Bibliography: p.
ISBN 0-7710-6065-3 (bound). – ISBN 0-7710-6069-6 (pbk.).

1. Parenting 2. Parent and child. 3. Children –
Management. I. Title.

HQ755.8.M56   649'.1   C82-094684-2

Printed and bound in Canada

Contents

Dedication

To Maxine
Whose love and belief made all things possible.

To Karen, Nancy, Marilyn, David, Harvey, Kaleb, Rachel,
Michael, and Elyse
Who have made all things worthwhile.

Acknowledgements

Of all the many roles I have played the best has been trying to be a father. It helped to have a supportive, enthusiastic wife and three daughters who were forgiving of errors and who cheered my successes.

As a researcher and practitioner I am grateful to the many parents and children I have counselled. They taught me much: I felt with them, sometimes cried with them, and became excited with their new skills and the resolution of their problems. Change is painful and change is slow but with good intention it happens.

To my colleagues, Dr. Leo Lazar, Dr. Bernice Mandelcorn, Dr. Harvey Mandel, Dr. Marc Wilcheski, Dr. Helen Doan, Dr. Shirley Stack, and Dr. Joe Willis my sincere appreciation for their unceasing enthusiasm and encouragement.

To Dr. Benjamin Spock, Dr. Carl Rogers, and Dr. Thomas Gordon for their example and inspiration.

To Beverley Slopen and Jack McClelland for their belief.

To Jean Christie, Jackie Roberge, Dianne Zecchino, Zehra Ali Khan, David Hellyer, Roberta Bucovetsky, and Dick and Laurna Tallman for their friendship, advice, and professional expertise.

I thank you.

Harold A. Minden

Preface:

What's the Best Book on Parenting?

In my practice as a psychologist, I am often asked this question. There is no "best book," and there probably never will be one single book that can answer all questions and solve all problems.

Parenting is a complex profession. And, as in all other professions, one needs a great deal of information, instruction, training, and more training to be good at it. Reading one book simply won't – by itself – do the job. You would hardly expect to become an outstanding teacher, or a surgeon, or an architect by reading a *single* book.

Yet, many authors who write on parenting write as if their book were the definitive, final word on parenting, an encyclopedia of everything one should know. Because of the complexity of the subject and the enormous range of differences in parents and children, and in their needs and circumstances, any book that sets out to cover everything ends up by treating the subject lightly and inadequately – a wide-band, low-fidelity treatment.

By contrast, certain writers, such as Spock, Briggs, Dodson, Ginott, Gordon, and Dreikers, do not attempt to be all things to all readers on child-rearing. They have specific messages, articulated with clarity, loaded with good examples, and written with sensitivity. So which should you read? All of them! Which should you follow? The answer depends on your needs and your style. It would be neat and tidy to find "the answer" from a single source. But parenting requires one to combine and adapt countless "bits" of information and counsel from numerous child-rearing experts.

Over a period of many years of practice in child psychology, I have counselled many children brought to me with learning, emotional, and behavioural problems. I would see a given child for perhaps one or two hours a week, while the child's mother sat in the waiting room thinking (1) "Whew, I feel better – it's not my problem for an hour or two"; or (2) "The 'expert' will help him." The flaw in this mother's thinking was her belief – her hope – that *anyone*, however expert, can cure *anything* in one hour a week without also working with and strengthening the parents so they can survive the other 167 hours in the week.

I came to recognize this weakness, so my focus and my procedures changed: I became "parent-oriented." I began to try to help parents to define their children's problems and to develop the skills required to solve them. Success was when the parents became the experts themselves, able to face and resolve their own dilemmas.

But even this new focus was not enough. I discovered that parents were having difficulties with their children because (1) the parents did not have their own act together as individuals, and (2) their marriages had unresolved problems of their own, and they lacked the skills to cope with them. Johnny's reading problem, for example, or his low self-esteem or aggressiveness was often the result of his parents' own low self-esteem and high anxiety and the climate of constant bickering in the home. Johnny's reading problem, or his self-esteem problems or his aggressiveness, cannot be treated effectively without also treating the whole environment in which it finds expression.

What this book has to say about learning, motivation, self-discipline, the infectiousness of failure, self-esteem, stress management, patience, communication, and the importance of love and affection is relevant to the development of the individual as an individual, as partner in marriage, and as parent. When we resolve our own personal and marriage problems, many of the concerns we have as parents will disappear on their own. If they do not, we will need to acquire additional understanding, special skills, and strategies to cope with them.

In a recent survey we conducted with hundreds of parents, 41 per cent of the participants reported that parenthood was, for them, a frustrating, negative experience. A much smaller number – only 22 per cent – reported they had found parenthood positive and fulfilling. The survey also disclosed that more than half of the parents who reported that "parenting was the pits" considered their marriages *unsatisfactory* or *very unsatisfactory*. By contrast, 79 per cent of the parents who found parenting fulfilling regarded their marriages as *satisfactory* or *very satisfactory*.

It is also significant that 61 per cent of the parents who considered parenting "frustrating" were concerned about their own lack of self-esteem and self-confidence. Conversely, 81 per cent of the fulfilled parents reported good to high self-esteem. These research findings corroborate what many clinical psychologists have learned in practice: that parents who like themselves are more likely to enjoy, and be good at, marriage and parenthood. Though specific information on the how and when of such learning as "potty training" is essential, an additional agenda also has to be attended to in order to avoid compounding the inevitable questions and problems of growing. If children have *any* rights, they have the right to parents who have acquired some knowledge and learned some parenting skills and who also feel good about themselves as individuals and as marriage partners.

These skills and this sense of self-worth are not the results solely of book learning. Courses and books are not by themselves the answer. They offer part of the information needed and just part of the answer. It's what you bring to the book learning that can make it valuable. Our parenting styles and attitudes are developed from the experiences we have had as children, from our parents, grandparents, and friends. Newspapers, magazines, movies, and television are always promoting what we should and should not be doing. Religious and societal values shape our values and needs.

The goodness of a good parenting book or course is not that it gives you a specific answer to every possible question but that it gives you some basic understanding of child development and some tools, skills, and strategies so that you are capable of dealing with and resolving the inevitable problems and hurdles in parenthood.

A parenting book can be a useful guide outlining various routes you can take and what you can expect along the journey. Such, it is my hope, is the present book, *Two Hugs for Survival*. It doesn't take you there nor does it guarantee what happens on arrival; it does seek to make the trip more enjoyable and less a matter of trial and error.

ONE

Where Did We Go Wrong?

The prevalent mythology of parenting in society is that it is a naturally acquired skill which, if properly applied, will produce beautiful, intelligent, fun-loving children who will bring joy, peace and contentment into the parents' lives. Reality contradicts that mythology.
— MICHAEL SMITH

I don't know that I have been a better father because of my training as a psychologist, but I do know that I am a more understanding psychologist because of my experiences as a father. This book is not only about the many children and the parents I have worked with professionally and about our parent-training workshops and our research findings; it is also about my own personal experiences as a father of three daughters, who I hope never felt they were subjects in a psychological experiment.

When the psychologist has a family there is a danger in identifying too closely with the problems presented by the parents who come for professional assistance. Fortunately, I had a very wise clinical professor who taught us well. He would caution us to be careful:

> There will be times in your professional career that you will be angry and frustrated and you will want to take every troubled kid home. Your first judgement may be that the child's condition is a result of an environment where the parents don't care, don't love, and are incapable of being adequate parents. You will be wrong since 95 per cent of our parents do care, do love, and have the potential to be effective parents.

The professor was right. There were times when I felt frustrated because it appeared that the parents were the cause of their child's problem. In most cases, however, I have found that the parents' behaviour was motivated by good intentions but questionable judgement.

The Case of Jamie T.

On one of my consultations at the hospital I met an old school friend I hadn't seen for over twenty years. He was waiting for the elevator but whenever it opened he would back away from it and not go in. He looked very distraught. As I approached him to say hello it occurred to me why he was in the hospital – it was his son who had been admitted for an overdose of drugs and was in a very serious condition. We sat and talked for over an hour. He was overcome with grief and guilt. He felt his stupidity and rigidity were the cause of his son's condition. "If only I could turn the clock back. If only I had another chance. I love that kid so much. We never understood Jamie. He was always the butt for everything that went wrong at home. Where did we go wrong?"

That night I talked with Jamie's mother, or rather, I listened. She had so much to say that had been bottled up for so long.

"Well, Jamie has forced us to stop playing our charade. Our life has been such a masquerade. To friends and outsiders we have been a model family. Our family problems were always well hidden or lied about. We all need help."

And through her tears she began to tell her story....

"I sat in the waiting room of the psychiatric ward and sobbed. My body, my head, my heart – everything hurt so badly. John sat hunched trying to muffle what he always had considered unmanly – crying. What we had just seen couldn't have happened to us. Our son, Jamie, whom we both loved, was lying in this hospital with a brain that has been severely damaged by an overdose of drugs. We were told that the prognosis for full recovery was questionable. We saw this pathetic, thin little figure lying in the intensive care unit with tubes and wires and incoherent babbles.

"I thought back seventeen years to the time we brought our first baby home from the hospital. What excitement! We had great plans and great expectations. He was going to be an excellent athlete, the valedictorian. He would go into engineering and then join his father's company. He was going to be a big success! We also secretly hoped that Jamie would help resolve the differences we were having in our marriage, which seemed to be a constant series of quarrels, skirmishes, battles, and peace treaties.

"Jamie was irritable and hyperactive from the very first month. He cried continuously and kept us up all night. John often moved down to the recreation room with 'I have to go to work tomorrow and I need my sleep.' For him, parenthood was motherhood – that's how it was in his parents' home. He would make me feel guilty if I asked him to hold Jamie or change him during the night in between feedings. There were nights when I was so sick and tired I could fall asleep standing up.

"Jamie didn't heal our marriage and I think we began to blame him and use him as a scapegoat for escalating our battles to a full-scale war. Our pediatrician said he would grow out of the hyperactivity, irritability, and mixed-up sleeping cycles. When Jamie finally went off to school, his teachers complained about his constant fidgeting, inattention, lying, and rudeness. We took him everywhere – to a psychiatrist, an allergist, a nutritionist, a pediatric neurologist. He was finally put on a heavy dose of Ritalin. While Jamie was being treated with an amphetamine my doctor prescribed Valium for my anxiety and nervous condition. John coped with his miseries with alcohol and silence.

"My in-laws fuelled the fires by comparing Jamie to their 'golden boy.' Their innuendos were a constant indictment of me for spoiling and indulging Jamie.

"We had another child, a little girl, Patricia, and she was almost everything Jamie wasn't. She was good at school, never got into any difficulties, matured and developed according to all of Dr. Spock's guidelines, but she always seemed distant and detached from the family. She was her own support system; never appeared to need encouragement, direction, or even a cuddle. She would disappear whenever there were family quarrels and we were so busy attacking or defending that I guess we welcomed her non-involvement – there were enough antagonists. She was our "star boarder." She kept everything neat, tidy, but separate – her things, her thoughts, her emotions, her friends, and her school life. My in-laws kept comparing Patricia to their son and were convinced that Patricia had inherited John's independence, diligence, neatness, control, and high need for personal privacy. When I think of Pat growing up, it was like ships passing in the night. We knew she was there but we didn't see her and our radar equipment showed no distress signals. Our radar was faulty.

"By the time Jamie turned sixteen he had a record, a bad record – at school and at home. The agenda of our whole life now seemed centred around this 'bad kid.' I seemed to have become a secondary adversary since the action was now between father and son. Jamie's long hair, patched jeans, and failures at school irritated and embarrassed his father. The battles became more and more intense, and when Jamie was caught smoking marijuana he was verbally and physically beaten and warned that if he was caught smoking again he would be kicked out of the house. That night, I think both Jamie and I cried ourselves to sleep.

"One month later, John kept his promise. He caught Jamie smoking grass in the laundry room. He grabbed him, hit him, threw him out, and told him he never wanted to see him again. John and I had our biggest quarrel that night and it ended up with John packing an overnight bag, grabbing a bottle, and leaving the house. My life seemed to be a complete disaster. I thought about divorce, suicide, or just running away. John and I got back together for a temporary truce, but it was a house where the three of us, John, Pat, and I, lived with only the minimum of communication. We each carried out our household responsibilities, but it was an empty, silent house.

"One year later we received an urgent call from the local hospital. 'Your son has been admitted to our psychiatric ward. Could you come right down?'

"When we arrived, before we were allowed to see Jamie, the attending physician wanted to talk to us. 'Your son has had a bad time and for a while we didn't think he would make it. He took enough LSD to kill him. There may be some brain damage. How much improvement there will be over time is anyone's guess. He babbles, he rocks, he cries. He's been this way for two weeks. What he needs now is a combination of our medical treatment and your love and affection. This is not the time to sit in judgement on what he has done. Just hold him and hug him. Be with him totally and if you know how to pray – pray for him.'

"Our war is over and like all wars there are no winners. Where did we go wrong?"

According to Dr. Sidney Jourard, sickness is often our final protest and a cry for help. Jamie's overdose was perhaps his way of saying, "I hurt so much inside. I don't know what to do or where to go!" And since no one listened and no one understood his pain and his failure, Jamie learned to escape his anguish with powders and pills.

Is this family really so unusual? Do they really differ from millions of other families, or are the casualties just heavier? Do these problems only happen to parents with deep emotional, psychological difficulties. Not really! Many parents can see something of themselves, their marriage, their parenting, or their own parents in this family.

Jamie's parents were not "disturbed" people. They both had strengths and special, endearing qualities. They entered marriage with deep feelings of love for each other and in their own style they loved Jamie and Patricia. What went wrong to all their hopes, good intentions, and love for each other? Why did life become a series of disagreements, arguments, resentment, and unhappiness? How could all of this have been prevented? Were Jamie's parents prepared for either marriage or parenthood? How many of us are?

A number of questions and observations present themselves from this brief case history.

- The parents came from quite different backgrounds and had a fixed pattern of lifestyles, habits, and expectations. Were they ever acknowledged or resolved? Did their differences become their strength or weakness?
- What did their marriage agreement or contract look like? Did they openly share their expectations of each other, their motives, and their needs?

- John's view of parenthood as being motherhood (as was the case in his family) – how might they have resolved this contentious view?
- Did they really understand child development? Was Jamie's hyperactivity an organic, constitutional problem or was it the result of their marriage distress? Was Jamie's condition irreversible? What skills did they need to cope with his difficulties other than always running to professionals to have him "doctored" and corrected?
- What about their expectation that having children would resolve their marital problems? Was this a reasonable motive for having children?
- Did John's use of physical punishment as a disciplinary measure help or did it create more casualties? Did it help the communication between John and Jamie? Did throwing Jamie out of the house lead to his drug addiction? What were the alternatives?
- The quarrels, the battles, the Ritalin, the Valium, and the alcohol did not resolve any of their problems but only compounded them. What were their options and what strategies could have helped them manage their stress and impatience?
- Patricia's silence, detachment, and extreme need for privacy – was this normal behaviour?
- How much time did Mother and Patricia spend together? Did they have a close one-to-one relationship? Or Jamie and Mother or Jamie and John? Did they take the time to be with each other, to listen, to share their ups and downs, their successes and failures, their thoughts, their ambitions? Did the parents have a good one-to-one relationship where they had time to share, plan, laugh, cry, and love each other? Or was the family agenda only one of blame, criticism, and invective?
- Bickering and quarreling are infectious – they create a climate for more disagreement and bad feeling. Conversely, love, a hug, affection, empathy, faith, and a supportive attitude can create a climate where parents and children can grow and enjoy each other.

In short, were the problems that this family experienced so abnormal?

After seeing many families in difficulty I began to wonder whether we were seeing a select group of problem families in our mental health clinics and private practice. Or were the difficulties similar but just more intense than in normal families? To answer this question we developed a survey and interviewed hundreds of parents. They reflected a wide sampling of different educational, religious, social, and economic backgrounds. We interviewed the married, the single parent, bank managers, teachers, mechanics, secretaries, physicians, salespeople, and housewives. What we found was, in many ways, a big surprise.

For 41 Per Cent, Parenting Is the Pits!

Survey Question 12

How would you rate your parenting experience?

[   ] Fulfilling and positive
[   ] Moderately fulfilling
[   ] Frustrating and negative

Results

22 per cent of the parents answered "fulfilling and positive."
37 per cent of the parents answered "moderately fulfilling."
41 per cent of the parents answered "frustrating and negative."

These were among the results obtained in our survey of hundreds of parents from different educational and ethnic backgrounds, religious affiliations, and economic circumstances. If these reactions reflect the experience of the general population, then there are approximately *thirty million* parents in North America who are having great difficulty and who have found parenting a "frustrating and negative experience." When one considers the nights and the days, the months and the years of time invested, and the physical, emotional, mental, and economic expenditures, the results are devastating. Perhaps what happens to the children of the *41 per cent* is even more serious.

These results raise a number of questions. What, for example, are the differences between the frustrated parents and the successful, fulfilled parents? What is one group doing that is so right and the other doing so badly? Do their differences have something to do with their maternal or paternal instincts, heredity, motivation, skills, training, or just plain luck?

A Comparative Profile: Fulfilled Parents and Frustrated Parents

From the enormous amount of data obtained from the hundreds of parents who co-operated in this survey, two very distinct profiles have emerged which indicate that the 22 per cent who found parenting to be "fulfilling and positive" differ radically in many particulars from the 41 per cent in the "frustrating and negative" category. Answers submitted dealt with their motivation for parenthood, their qualifications, their preparation for parenthood, their parenting styles, the condition of their marriage, their level of patience and stress, and their personal self-esteem. These were some of the dramatic differences:

In our Motivation for Parenthood Test, which was developed by a panel of parents, the "fulfilled" group scored significantly higher on the "positive motives" and the "frustrated" scored higher on the "negative motives" for wanting children. The 22 per cent decided to because they loved children, enjoyed the company of children, felt capable of being parents, and were excited about having, teaching, and caring for children. On the other hand, many of the 41 per cent gave answers like these as their reasons for having children:

- "It's just expected of you when you get married."
- "To keep my marriage together."
- "It's a moral obligation."
- "Having kids removes any doubts about my sexual adequacy."
- "My kids will achieve the success I never had the opportunity for."
- "I'm lonely."
- "Pressure from my parents or friends."

Though many factors besides the initial motives for having children will influence how effective parents will be, the parents' original motives give important clues to their probabilities for success – or failure – in parenting.

TABLE 1

Preparation for Parenthood

	the 22% Successful Parents	*the 41%* Frustrated Parents
Had attended lectures or courses on parenting or child development	64%	19%
Mothers had read one or more books on parenting	89%	37%
Fathers had read one or more books on parenting	41%	7%
Felt qualified and capable as a parent	76%	29%

It's obvious from the above findings that there is a critical difference between the "successful" and the "frustrated" in their preparation for parenthood. Parenting is a difficult and intricate profession for which a parent needs training if serious problems are to be avoided. Parent education may not eliminate all problems but it may help in understanding and resolving them.

An additional finding of importance: while 69 per cent of the successful parents said they would enrol in additional courses on parenting if they were offered, only 37 per cent of the frustrated parents would do so. It would appear that even though the "frustrated" are experiencing great difficulty, they do not recognize their need for assistance in parenting.

AN IRONIC TWIST

Question 41 – Do you think parents should be required to take courses in "How to Parent"? Of the frustrated parents, 61 per cent answered *yes*, that such courses should be mandatory, yet only 25 per cent of the "successful" felt that parents should be compelled to enrol in such training. It's as if the frustrated were saying: "Parent training is good and necessary. But I'll take the training only if it's compulsory and I am forced to enrol. I don't have the self-motivation or self-discipline to enrol on my own."

Personality Differences

SELF-ESTEEM AND SELF-CONFIDENCE

In the parent survey, 81 per cent of the successful parents rated their self-esteem *good* to *very high*, while only 39 per cent of the frustrated parents reported good or higher self-esteem. Substantial research evidence indicates that the way a child views himself or herself is strongly related to the self-concept of the child's mother or father. Self-esteem is contagious. Our findings appear to say that the children of frustrated parents will end up with the same poor self-concepts their parents have suffered.

SELF-CONTROL

Though approximately 80 per cent of both groups indicated that the one additional skill they needed most to cope with the problems of parenthood was *patience*, it turned out that the frustrated parents lost control and used physical punishment more often than their successful counterparts.

STRESS AND COPING STRATEGIES

Information drawn from the survey does not allow us to assume that individuals were highly stressed before they became parents or that they became highly stressed because of parenthood. It does, however, indicate that the two groups are experiencing different levels of stress and reacting differently to stressful situations and their causes.

Frustrated parents reported much higher levels of stress in their lives, with child-behaviour problems, marriage difficulties, shortage of time, fatigue, and impatience as the most critical causes of stress. They also coped differently, smoking, drinking, and eating more than the successful group. Twenty-six per cent of the frustrated parents reported taking tranquilizers regularly and were less frequently involved in physical and recreational activity, such as sports, music, and hobbies, than the parents who were enjoying their parenting role.

Though there wasn't a difference between the two groups in the use of prayer for stress reduction, there was a significant difference in their ability to share and discuss their stress with their spouses or friends.

STATE OF MARRIAGE

It appears that many of the frustrated parents are also unhappy and frustrated in marriage. Fifty-two per cent of these parents rated their marriage from unsatisfactory to very unsatisfactory, whereas 79 per cent of the successful parents rated their marriage satisfactory or better.

The frustrated parents reported poor communication with their spouse and the mothers in this group complained about the lack of fathers' sharing of responsibility for parenting. The reports from the successful parents, on the other hand, suggested they have a good partnership and that it takes a father's involvement to make parenting more fulfilling. There is a strong relationship between this lack of the father's involvement and the stress level, the irritability, and impatience that the mother experiences.

Though the data from this study is correlational and does not give evidence of cause and effect, it does suggest that parents should work out their marriage problems before having children, since the problems are compounded with the added responsibility for children. Many of the frustrated parents reported that having children "put a strain on their marriage." Conversely, most of the successful parents reported that their children had "improved and enriched" their marriages.

Child-rearing Styles

The differences between the two groups in terms of child-rearing practices are dramatic.

COMMUNICATION

They differ significantly in their levels of communication with their children, their spouses, and specifically in their one-to-one relationships with their children. Seventy-seven per cent of the successful parents indicated they had one-to-one relationships with their children. They spent time (on an individual basis) talking, working, learning, and playing together. Only 18 per cent of the frustrated parents had established such one-to-one relationships with their children.

DISCIPLINE AND PUNISHMENT

The groups were also disparate in their attitudes toward discipline. The frustrated parents defined discipline as a method of punishment and control, but for many of the successful group, discipline meant "to educate." Though the frustrated parents used more physical punishment, they also reported that it was not very effective. The successful parents usually resorted to discussion, reason, and loss of privileges as disciplinary measures.

FATHER'S INVOLVEMENT

The successful group of fathers spent more time with their children each day. They read to them, played with them, listened to them, put them to bed, and had good one-to-one relationships with their children. They were committed and involved fathers and were not, as Margaret Mead described fathers, "biological necessities but social accidents."

AFFECTION

Successful parents were much more affectionate toward their children than the frustrated parents. Their style of affection included a lot of physical contact (hugging; an arm around the shoulder; and hello, good-bye, or goodnight kisses), such verbal declarations as "I like you" or "I love you," joking, teasing, and playing with them. As one parent stated, "I think my affection for my children is written in the smile all over my face."

TWO-PARENT FAMILIES VS. SINGLE-PARENT FAMILIES

The findings reported so far were derived from two-parent families. When we compared single-parent to two-parent families, several significant differences surfaced. Take, for example, the answers of single parents to this question: How would you describe your parenting experience? Results:

32 per cent reported "fulfilling and positive."
22 per cent reported "moderately fulfilling."
46 per cent reported "frustrating and negative."

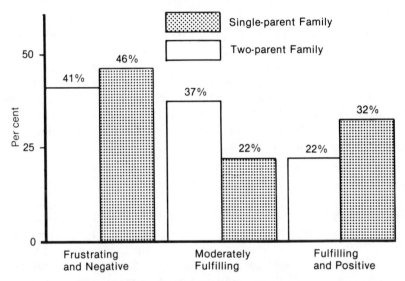

Figure 1. The Parenting Experience

It appears that the experiences of single parents are rather more extreme than those of two-parent families. They are either *very good* or *very bad*, and not as much in between. Whereas only 22 per cent of the two-parent families reported success in parenting, 32 per cent of the single parents reported that their parenting experiences have been "fulfilling and positive." And where 41 per cent of the two-parent families found parenting frustrating, greater numbers of the single-parent family – 46 per cent – reported parenting was a "frustrating and negative" experience.

The survey disclosed that single parents take fewer courses but read more books on parenting. They spend more time doing things with their children on a one-to-one basis. They report more stress in their lives, but the causes of stress they list are less child-oriented than those of the two-parent families. Single parents listed such sources of stress as loneliness, finances, irritability, tiredness, and a lack of adult conversation, company, and sex. They use more cigarettes, alcohol, drugs, and professional help to cope with their stress. One interesting finding was that more single parents than two-parent families would have children if they had the choice to make again. In one other significant comparison, both the successful and frustrated single parents were similar to their two-parent counterparts: patience was the skill both agreed that they needed to develop.

A Package of Problems

From the evidence at hand, it appears that the frustrated-parent group has a "package of problems," starting with love and self-esteem and extending on through marriage difficulties. The problems are compounded by their lack of preparation and training for the most difficult of professions – parenthood. Parents probably would not let an untrained mechanic repair their car, yet many tinker, without preparation, with the most complex system in the world – the physical, emotional, intellectual, spiritual, and social well-being of their children.

THE OBVIOUS IS NOT ALWAYS SO OBVIOUS

Did we really need to run this extensive study? Shouldn't it be obvious to everyone that successful parents "have their act together," that they like themselves, enjoy their marriage, have taken the time to prepare themselves for parenting, and are enjoying their children? Yet, if all this is so obvious, why haven't the frustrated 41 per cent examined their motives for parenthood, their qualifications, their preparation, their own personalities, and the states of their marriages? The consequence of their frustration is costly, in terms of what happens to their children.

Did differences in education, religion, or income distinguish the successful from the unsuccessful parents? No – none of these factors differentiated the two groups. Nor did marital status make a major difference. There actually was a higher percentage of single parents who found parenting "fulfilling and positive." As for education levels and incomes, there were college graduates with incomes over $30,000 per year and drop-outs and low-income families in both groups.

TWO

Successful Parenting:

Instinct, Heredity, Skill, or Luck?

Child-rearing is not usually regarded as a professional skill for which people need to be selected, trained or paid for. It is, however, as difficult and intricate as any profession. Training of parents in child-rearing would be one of the best ways of preventing delinquency and mental disorder.

— PROFESSOR MICHAEL ARGYLE, OXFORD UNIVERSITY

Is there any other occupation in the world on which everyone is prepared to embark without training, without experience and without any more specialized knowledge than is provided by having been, so to speak, on the receiving end a good many years before? An occupation which will affect the health and happiness if not the actual survival of one or more people, I am referring of course to the job of being parent which most of us undertake so lightheartedly and which for most of us again, turns out to be so different from anything we expected. Our surprise takes innumerable and varied forms, some pleasant, some disagreeable.

— CATHERINE STORR

Am I Responsible for All of This Child?

This is the question, and the lament, of many parents. And the answer is *NO* – not all, but *most* of him (or her). Over and beyond the parents' involvement, there are many other factors that can influence a child's development, such as the child's genetic inheritance, state of health, brothers, sisters, grandparents, the extended family, friends, teachers and the educational system, societal attitudes, laws, and opportunities. The parents are, however, the *first* and *most influential* of all the factors. Parents are the child's first providers of all basic needs, such as love,

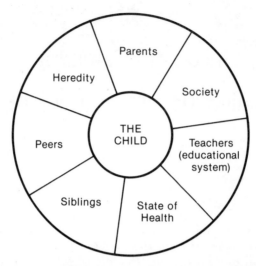

Figure 2. Factors that Influence a Child's Growth and Development

physical affection, feeding, bathing, and changing, and they are the child's first and most important teachers and models. The foundations for language, self-concept, emotional stability, and physical and mental growth are laid down by the parents.

Maternal and Paternal Instincts?

More than 32 per cent of the parents in our survey believe that parenting is instinctive. They believe that maternal and paternal instincts motivate them to have children in the first place. They also believe that the abilities to understand and to raise children are instinctive. Birds do it and bees do it instinctively, so why not humans?

Theorists and researchers from many disciplines have debated the phenomenon of instinct for years. An instinct is defined as a behaviour that is *not* learned, is universal, and is there at birth. Some instinct theorists have suggested that we are born with as many as a thousand instincts, ranging from an instinct for hoarding to an instinct for aggression, and that most of our behaviour is determined by instincts. Empirical evidence over the years has debunked most of the instinct claims. A few cling tenaciously, including the most widely held of all – the maternal instinct.

But there is controversy as to whether humans inherit any maternal or paternal instincts at all. Erik Erikson suggests that becoming a parent is an expression of an *innate motivation* to care for and teach the young.

Erich Fromm refers to the innate quality of a mother's "unconditional love." Though there may be this instinct to want children and to love and take care of them, there is strong evidence that disproves the notion that parenting *skills* are instinctive. To this scientific evidence we should add the millions of messed-up kids and the high incidence of child punishment and abuse. If there is such a thing as a maternal or paternal instinct, either it's not enough to cope with the complexity of human existence or – in the process of evolution – it is disappearing.

The message is clear for the 32 per cent who believe in instincts – don't depend on them!

How Influential Are Parents in Child Development?

The parent survey reported in the previous chapter focused primarily on parents' feelings, problems, experiences, training, and attitudes and did not directly examine children's experiences. There is an assumption here that seems logical: that parents are satisfied with their parenting abilities when a child is happy, well-adjusted, and functioning physically, socially, intellectually, and emotionally in an effective manner. The successful 22 per cent clearly identified themselves as the agents primarily responsible for a positive outcome. So the corollary question arises: when the outcome is negative are the frustrated 41 per cent responsible?

THE CELDIC REPORT

For three years, a group of professionals in Canada conducted an in-depth survey of children, parents, and services. They travelled widely, questioned, listened, poked, and probed. And what they found gave them much concern and "gave us much to make us weep."

They reported that 21 per cent of the population up to nineteen years of age, or no less than one million children (multiply this by ten to arrive at a U.S. equivalent) in Canada, require attention, treatment, and care because of emotional, behavioural, and learning disorders. Though they take issue with the professionals, they see the family environment – the parents – as the *most significant* influence in a child's formative years.

Parents are the key figures in setting the emotional climate for the child's growth. Their happiness or unhappiness, adjustment or mal-adjustment, their maturity, their relationship with one another, their satisfaction and enjoyment in this parental role will have profound consequences for the child's mental health and for his viability in the world outside the family. In most cases of children with adjustment or behaviour problems, the *root* of the difficulty seems to stem from disturbances in early relationships and family upbringing. (p. 31)

Studies in England, France, and the United States report similar findings with regard to the millions of children who have emotional, behavioural, and learning problems and are in need of professional help. According to Melanie Klein, between 1966 and 1971 alone there was a 63 per cent increase in the number of children being treated at one mental health facility. She concludes "that raising a child, especially today, is a worrisome business" and "that there are many times when parents will be the cause of their children's pain." Klein makes another important statement: "No one is more important in a child's life than his mother and father.... At the same time, parents should rid themselves of the oppressive sense that they alone are responsible for a child's emotional pain."

Anthony Storr of Oxford University points out that "Although most people would probably agree that the family is the best milieu in which to rear children, it must be recognized that home can be a dangerous place ... we like to think of the family as the abode of love, of home as the safe retreat where a child is sure of support and protection. The reality is often rather different."

There have been literally thousands of psychological studies on the effects of parents and child-rearing practices on a child's motor, sensory-motor, physical, intellectual, emotional, social, and ethical behaviour. Studies on the relationships between parent behaviour and language development, attention span, achievement motivation, anxiety, neurosis, delinquency, and attitudes toward politics, prejudice, eating, TV watching, and sex have been reported in the scientific journals.

Though many of these studies do not give us firm conclusions, they give us important guidance on effective and ineffective parenting styles and offer substantial evidence that parents are "the number one" influences, teachers, and shapers in a child's history – for the good and for the bad.

Research Findings on Parenting and Children's Behaviour

Research Report 1 (S. Coopersmith)
Children who are brought up under strongly structured conditions with specified limits tend to have a higher self-esteem and are more independent and creative than children reared in a permissive environment.

Research Report 2 (S. Coopersmith)
Children reared with definite limits are more socially acceptable, are capable of expressing their opinions, and can cope with criticism.

Research Report 3 (S. Coopersmith)
Children in families where there was marital tension expressed more anger outside the home, were very frustrated, and had lower self-esteem.

Research Report 4 (R. Sears)
Maternal and paternal warmth and acceptance are directly related to a child's self-esteem.

Research Report 5 (E.R. Lanza)
An affectionate, harmonious marriage resulted in children with good to high self-confidence and self-esteem.

Research Report 6 (S. Jourard)
"If you like your parents you tend to be like them." Children's self-concepts resemble their parents' self-concepts.

Research Report 7 (S. Minuchin)
Marital difficulties limit a child's potential for emotional growth.

Research Report 8 (R. Sears, E. Maccoby, and H. Levin)
Harsh physical punishment at home was equated with high childhood aggressiveness at school.

Research Report 9 (M. Radke)
Children from restrictive homes in which punishment was severe and control autocratic had more problems with teachers and peers.

Research Report 10 (E. Bing)
The level of parental language stimulation and comprehensive verbal explanation was related to children's intellectual development and language ability.

Research Report 11 (H. Mussinger)
Punishing parents produce dependent, inhibited, withdrawn children who have great difficulty in adjusting to school and later life in the community. Children of parents who are loving but controlling produce children who are submissive, dependent, have poor social skills, and are not very creative.

Research Report 12 (W. Becker)
Parents who use withdrawal of love as punishment have children who are anxious, feel guilty, and suffer from low self-concept.

Research Report 13 (R. Blanchard and H. Biller)
Families where the father was absent frequently had children with lower cognitive skills and more emotional and behavioural problems.

Research Report 14 (J. Kagan and K. Moss)
Parental encouragement and warmth were related to high achievement motivation in children.

Research Report 15 (J. Bigner)
Children who lack a fathering experience have problems in the area of personality and social development.

Research Report 16 (E. Hetherington)
A father's absence creates difficulties for adolescent girls in their ability to relate to male peers.

Research Report 17 (J. Piaget)
Parental prohibitions against exploration and curiosity can result in children with learning problems and slower intellectual development.

Research Report 18 (R. Hess and V. Shipman)
The potential for mental growth, language abilities, and academic achievement is influenced strongly by a mother's language-teaching style.

The above studies are but a small sample of the evidence that relates parent behaviour to child behaviour and may well be used an an index of do's and don'ts. Perhaps one of the most instructive research studies was carried out by Diana Baumrind, who identified three different parenting styles: the *authoritative parent*, the *authoritarian parent*, and the *permissive parent*. Authoritative parents are firm but warm, non-rejecting, consistent, willing to explain and reconsider rules. Their children are the most competent, self-reliant, self-controlled, and content. Authoritarian parents are detached, highly controlling, restrictive, over-protective, and unwilling to discuss or reconsider rules. Their children are less competent, more discontent, withdrawn, and distrustful. Permissive parents are non-controlling and non-demanding and establish no firm rules. Their children are the least competent and the most dependent, aimless, and irresponsible.

Baumrind's research indicates that the attributes of competence, independence, outgoingness, self-control, and self-reliance are fostered by supportive home environments in which independent actions and decision-making as well as responsible and self-reliant behaviour are modeled, encouraged, and rewarded. Authoritative parents, who combine high but reasonable maturity demands, clearly defined standards of behaviour with open communication, and explanations of the reason for these standards, promote the development of mature, competent, and socially responsible children. Notedly, these parents do not use arbitrarily authoritarian discipline, severe punitiveness, and overprotection.

How do these research studies, which investigate specific areas of parent and child behaviour, relate to what is happening generally in society? How can they be used to reverse the trend toward increased learning, emotional, and delinquency problems, and what direction do they give us toward lessening the difficulties and complexities of our society (for example, the 40-50 per cent rate of separation, divorce, and broken homes)?

Even though, as was indicated by a District of Columbia Court of Appeals, "What a child needs is not a mother, but someone who can provide mothering," at this point in time it is the parent who has this responsibility. And there is strong evidence that some parents are either not prepared for this responsibility or do not choose to accept it.

Is It Heredity or Environment?

From the above research, one might gain the impression that a child's parents and his environment are *solely* responsible for his present and future personality and behaviour. This impression would be incorrect.

Heredity is an important factor – the product depends on the material you have to work with. There are great differences of opinion today as to the relative influences of heredity and environment. We have moved away from the early era in the history of child study when it was believed that "you are what your genes are." In other words, your intellectual level, personality, and physical self were thought to be predetermined totally by your genetic inheritance. This was followed by an era when orthodox environmentalists claimed that genes may determine certain physical characteristics, but all else is determined by your environment. Today, the accepted position is that *both* genes and environment are important, and that the real question is not how much each contributes, but *how* they interact and how the genes affect a specific psychological behaviour.

Our genes influence environmental factors, and environmental factors influence inheritance – and this interaction is constant. For example, if a child is born educably retarded (a condition which may be determined by his genes), and if his parents (who are his environment) reject the child and keep him closeted or send him to an institution, they have put a ceiling on the development of whatever intellectual equipment the child has inherited. Thus, he will never reach his potential. A child's environment can reduce him to a non-functioning human being, or – conversely – make him a human being who can learn and perform a great number of behaviours, who can love and give his family a sense of warmth and fulfilment.

A child may inherit great musical ability. Whether he or she becomes a concert pianist may be predetermined by environmental opportunities. On the other hand, a child born with less talent may be exposed to an exciting and encouraging environment and may reach high levels of achievement. The interaction of heredity and environment is an interplay of many complex variables.

What characteristics are inherited and how can parents best encourage and bring to fruition a child's genetic potential? There is strong evidence, based on the study of identical twins, that suggests our genes determine, to a great extent, our physical maturation, stature, appearance, intellectual potential, musical and artistic potential, predisposition to disease (for example, diabetes, asthma, allergies, and heart function). The same studies also suggest that our genes determine a number of personality characteristics.

Genes and Personality

THE INHERITANCE OF INTROVERSION AND EXTROVERSION

Research on the genetics of personality suggests that there is a hereditary component in "sociability." That is, whether you are an introvert – shy, withdrawn, timid – or an extrovert – self-confident, gregarious, friendly, active, and outgoing – is partially predetermined by your genes. The research also demonstrates that the introversion-extroversion sociability trait appears to be stable over many years. However, an enriched environment can modify and help an introverted child to become more outgoing and friendly. Conversely, a deprived environment can submerge or redirect an extroverted personality into submission or regression.

THE NEED FOR STIMULATION, CHANGE, AND ACTIVITY

A second personality trait linked to genetic factors is the individual's need and preference for different types and amounts of stimulation. Some children prefer an environment full of excitement and great change; others are disturbed by too many changes, too much sound, and too many new sights or people.

ACTIVITY NEEDS

Strong evidence suggests that our need for physical activity is also influenced by hereditary factors; and that, like sociability, this characteristic is relatively stable from the foetal stage to adolescent activity. Children with a high need for activity also demonstrate more irritability, are more impulsive, and encounter more difficulties in their early adjustment. It takes special parenting skills to channel this need into productive activity and learning.

CUDDLERS AND NON-CUDDLERS

The need for physical contact, cuddling, and gentling is an inherited trait. There seems to be a wide variation in this need. Some infants and young children are cuddlers and are soothed by hugs and physical comforting; others, the non-cuddlers, are more readily settled down by being rocked, walked, or sung to. The non-cuddlers are often more irritable, impulsive, restless, and physically active, but they can change depending on the parental treatment they receive.

THE INHERITANCE OF ANXIETY

A number of research studies in different countries have given us additional evidence of the genetic factors in thrill-seeking, neurosis, delinquency, and psychopathy. Studies by Professor Eysenck of the University of London report that 50 per cent of your level of anxiety is determined by heredity. That is, your genes determine to a great extent whether you are going to be an anxious or calm individual. This is an important finding, and parents need to develop an ability to read this predisposition to anxiety, and then to provide the anxious child with coping skills.

Temperaments from Birth: Three Types of Infants

Additional evidence on the role of heredity in personality is provided by three physicians, Alexander Thomas, Stella Chess, and Herbert G. Birch. Observing youngsters over a period of years, they encountered reasons "to question the prevailing one-sided emphasis on environment." They saw children with severe psychological difficulties who were living in family environments similar to those of children who had no problems. They also found that family disorganization and poor parental treatment were not, by themselves, adequate evidence on which to base a prediction of a child's future. They came to the conclusion that the variable omitted in any prediction was the temperament inherited by the child at birth. From their observations, they concluded that, to understand a child's personality, we must take into account the *interaction* of heredity and environment.

They investigated this concept by observing 141 children from infancy for about fourteen years. From in-depth and regular observations and detailed interviews with parents, they identified nine characteristics in children that could be discernible from the age of two to three months. These characteristics were found to be constant in a wide range of different population samples.

1. Level and amount of motor activity.
2. Regularity of such functions as eating, and the sleeping and wakefulness cycles.
3. The approach to or avoidance of new objects or persons.
4. Adaptability to changes in the child's environment.
5. Sensitivity to stimuli.
6. Level of intensity of the child's responses.
7. General mood (examples: cheerful, crying, cranky, or friendly).
8. Distractibility levels.
9. Attention span and persistence in activity.

From frequent parent interviews, home and school observations, teacher interviews, and psychological tests from infancy through pre-school, nursery, and elementary school, this trio of medical doctors concluded that "children do show distinct individuality in temperament in the first weeks of life *independent* of parent's handling or personality style. Our long-term study has now established that the original characteristics of temperament tend to persist over the years."

When Doctors Thomas, Chess, and Birch analysed the behavioural profiles of the 141 children in their test group they found that these nine characteristics clustered together. From these clusters there emerged three different types of personalities: the easy child, the difficult child, and the slow-to-warm-up child.

THE EASY CHILD

This child is characterized by positive moods, regularity in bodily functions, low intensity of reactions, adaptability, and easy approach to (rather than withdrawal from) new situations and people. The "easy infant" becomes the easy child, adapting to school and participating in new activities. Forty per cent of all the children they studied were easy children.

THE DIFFICULT CHILD

This child's native temperament includes irregular bodily functions, intensity of response, withdrawal when faced with new stimuli, slow adaptability, and negativity in mood. Difficult children cry a great deal, are often frustrated, and fly into temper tantrums. They have great difficulty in adjusting to new foods, people, routines, or activities. Ten per cent of the children in the studies could be placed in this category.

These children have a low need for motor activity, are slow to adapt, withdraw, are negative in mood, and have a quiet response to situations. Fifteen per cent of children studied were in this category.

The survey's results show that 65 per cent of the children could be placed categorically in one or another of the three categories, while 35 per cent had a mixture of traits. The danger with categories is that they can be too rigid. Also, they can be misused, since many children may fall into one category at one age and into another at another age. Or they may show some of the "symptoms" of the "easy child" and some of the "difficult child." Nonetheless, this work indicates that these are the predominant personality styles at birth and that they are consistent over the years of development. But they do voice a caveat: "Not all children in our study have shown a basic constancy of temperament, and inconsistency in temperament is itself a basic characteristic in some children."

What Can Parents Do About Heredity?

Doctors Thomas, Chess, and Birch point out that detailed knowledge of a child's temperamental characteristics can be extremely useful to parents in planning child-rearing practices and in guiding their own reactions to everyday situations. This understanding of a child's basic temperament is important both at home and at school. A child with a need for much activity should not be required to sit for long periods of time without some change or relief. If there is no opportunity for him to stretch, move, or expend his energy in a positive way, he often becomes labelled the *hyperactive child* and the "bad kid." The authors of this study conclude that it is important for parents to observe, understand, and accept these temperamental characteristics. But accepting them does not mean that there should be no attempt to create an environment that will modify negative traits and engender the growth of positive traits. Traits inherited at birth are not immutable: *they can be modified.*

These studies on the genetic basis of personality, intelligence, and physical functioning are important because they underscore the fact that parents are not responsible for *all* of what a child or adolescent is or becomes. Parents must, of course, be sensitive to a child's inherited temperament and capacities, since they are prime influences. Parenting behaviour can determine whether an "easy child" develops a negative personality marred by high anxiety and low self-esteem. Conversely, with patience, encouragement, and the application of sound parenting skills, a "difficult child" can become adaptable and self-confident about approaching new situations and learning social skills.

The data reported above indicate that we must take heredity into account, but that what finally happens to this inheritance will depend on the environment. *The environment.* In the child's most critical and formative years, the parents *are* its environment! How do their personalities, their attitudes, their understanding of child-rearing, and their skills affect the outcome? What type of parent promotes healthy development in a child, and what training does a parent need to create this healthy environment? The difference between the 22 per cent of parents who reported parenting as enjoyable and the 41 per cent for whom parenting was frustrating and negative, as discussed in Chapter One, can shed important light on these questions.

WHAT ARE YOUR CREDENTIALS?

What skills, what understanding, what licence do you have to be a prime agent, responsible for the most complex of all organisms and systems in this world? Human development is infinitely more complex than any computer, spaceship, or nuclear power plant.

For most of us it is "by guess or by God," by our own upbringing and a belief in instinct. All of the above are important influences, but they are not sufficient by themselves. With these credentials alone, you should not be allowed to tinker or teach very much. You are not allowed to tinker with, repair, or operate many of our mechanical systems without a licence earned through years of training; and even with years of training and retraining there are accidents. Yet without a day of training, without one course in parenthood, millions of men and women become the agents most responsible for raising a child, with all his complexities, in a complex and demanding world.

DO WE LACK THE TECHNOLOGY FOR SUCCESSFUL PARENTING?

According to the Celdic Report, we already possess an enormous body of information about development, and this scientific knowledge is being used neither appropriately nor adequately. There are four basic reasons why this knowledge is not properly exploited. (1) Parents have abdicated their responsibility for child-rearing to physicians, to psychologists, to government, and – perhaps most notable – to the child's teacher. Some parents expect teachers to be surrogate everythings. (2) Many professionals seek to assume the "Almighty Role" as respects their expertise in child-rearing. The Celdic Commission states that "No single factor caused us more concern than the picture of different professionals struggling to establish their own power base, distrustful of each other, refusing to share and so frequently failing the child." (3) Parents often have been relegated to a secondary or non-role; professionals have ignored parental effects, parental strengths, and parental weaknesses. (4) Much of our knowledge has not been translated into programs and then supplied to parents. These factors and the other research findings discussed here lead us to four basic commandments for successful parenting.

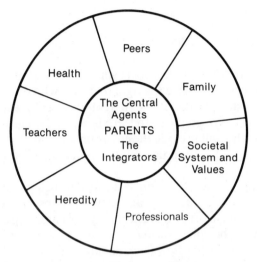

Figure 3. You Must Learn to Be Numero Uno

THE FOUR COMMANDMENTS

1. Parents must assume the central role for the care and management of their children. That role includes being a teacher, playmate, model, disciplinarian, listener, administrator, banker, ombudsman, and above all, a supplier of hugs, affection, and love.

2. Parents must recognize the role of teachers, physicians, and psychologists, and encourage the involvement of professionals, friends, siblings, and society. But they must not abdicate the central role to anyone, above all, not in the early, formative years.

3. Parenting is *not* instinctive. To be effective and comfortable in the role, you must take time to learn (a) to develop an understanding of children's needs and of the stages and phases of your child's growth and development, and (b) to develop a set of attitudes and skills that will make parenting effective and pleasurable for both you and your child. We rely too much on trial and error. We need, instead, training and instruction.

4. Finally, growth, development, and learning are not just for children. There is fun, excitement, and pain in growing together. The mistakes you make will not be fatal so long as the intent is to love and learn.

Children are very resilient. A dangerous assumption often made is that our role as parents is to insulate and shield our children from our mistakes and from the problems of life. Childhood isn't always happy-hood. We should never attempt to eliminate all bumps and disappointments. Children learn by owning and overcoming their own problems.

Conclusion: Children's Rights

Children don't have the right to decide whether they want to come into this world, and they don't have the right to decide who their parents are going to be. They do have the right to parents who really want them and love them, and who are prepared to learn how children grow. Children deserve parents who will provide the environment and opportunities to help them to grow and to capitalize on their potential. *Children have the right to qualified parents.*

The following chapters focus on well-tested principles and strategies that were developed in fifteen years of workshops and courses for parents. They should assist you in enjoying your parenting experiences. They also describe the child-rearing styles of the 22 per cent who were successful parents and offer further explanation for why the 41 per cent had problems.

THREE

Two Hugs for Survival

The importance of physical contact between mother and newborn child has been endorsed by the American Academy of Pediatrics and the American College of Obstetrics and Gynecology.
— NEWSPAPER REPORT

And the simple truth is that love cannot be assumed.... Children especially need a great deal of recognition and reaffirmation of their family's love for them. So parents who often find themselves saying in wonderment "Of course I love you, I'm your father" need to make their love more tangible. The testimony of love is not necessary through words, gifts or toys or material things but often more effectively through talking to or better yet listening to the children and finding ways to provide the humor, warmth, and affection as well as the guidance and direction they need.
— THOMAS MCGUINESS AND WILLIAM GLASER

My first assignment as a graduate student in psychology was to work with Professor Mortimer Appley, a noted researcher on stress. Dr. Appley was studying the effects of stress on emotional and learning behaviour and on physiological systems. I was delighted, since the assignment was regarded by students as a real plum.

What I *didn't* know was that the subjects in Dr. Appley's research study were Wistar rats. My first responsibility was to weigh each of the twenty-four rats used in his experiments, every day. I had never worked with rats; the thought of handling them gave me the shivers. I was instructed to pick them up by the neck, barehanded, and to weigh them on the lab scale.

When I opened the first rat cage to begin the weighing procedure, the rat backed into the corner and reared up on its haunches, forelegs wildly pawing the air. It appeared angry and vicious, and stared at me with a look that said, "Just put your hand in this cage and I'll tear it off." I quickly closed the cage door. My feelings were mixed: I was both scared of this little monster and angry with myself for being so afraid. I had watched other research assistants go through this routine daily, and it didn't seem to bother them.

That night my sleep was restless, filled with nightmares of giant, hungry rats. I decided to resign from the project because I just didn't have the guts to tangle with the rats. On my way to Dr. Appley's office to announce my resignation, I met Ken, a fellow graduate student, and told him my tale of woe. Ken suggested that, before I resigned, we should go together to the lab, check the animals, and he would show me how to work with them. Ken confided that he had had the same frightening experience in his first encounters with lab rats and that he had gradually overcome his fears. In the lab, Ken opened one cage – a rat literally "flew" out the door. For five minutes Ken chased the creature around the lab, at last catching it by its tail and tossing it back into its cage. "These animals are wild," he said. "You can't work with them." He asked me how old they were and if they had ever been gentled. ("Gentling" is a term used to describe the stroking and holding of newborn animals.)

It turned out the animals were ninety days old, which is late adulthood for rats, and that they had never been touched ... or gentled. According to Ken, these animals were wild and unmanageable because they had never been stroked or held.

I reported the condition of the animals – and my stark fear – to Professor Appley, and requested transfer to another research project involving (I hoped) "gentle humans." With great wisdom, the professor talked me into staying. "Animal behaviour parallels human behaviour," he said. "Our basic needs for food, water, and gentling are the same. You may have learned from this experience about one of life's greatest stressors – the absence of gentling."

Dr. Appley counselled me not to quit because of my fear. He suggested, instead, that I begin again with infant rats, nine to ten days old, assuring me these rats would be different. My instructions were to take them out of their cages each day, to hold, gentle, feed, and weigh them, and to observe the differences in their emotional reactions as compared to the ninety-day-old animals which had never been touched. So every day I gentled these soft, white, furry animals. They were playful, active, and docile, and enjoyed the physical handling. They became pets, and I began to give them names and to recognize that each of them was individual. The daily gentling made the difference between a terrorizing nightmare and an enjoyable adventure.

It was a dramatic lesson that I never forgot. In later years, as I began to work with retarded children and with neurologically handicapped and emotionally disturbed children and their parents, I began to witness sad evidence of this same lack of gentling. *There is a basic instinctual need in all humans for physical comforting,* and many of the children who were deprived of affectionate handling – especially in cases where the only contact was physical abuse – were like the animals: apprehensive, angry, disturbed, and sometimes even wild.

Physical Affection and the Human Child

It would be incorrect to assume that a mother's love and physical affection can cure all of society's ills, as Jean Jacques Rousseau once suggested, since there are other factors that influence the development of a healthy personality. But affection creates the basic climate needed for growth.

The importance of physical contact has been well-documented by the studies of Harry Harlow at the University of Wisconsin. Harlow used monkeys in his studies and discovered that severe emotional trauma resulted in infant monkeys when they were separated from their mothers soon after birth. Absence of direct physical contact with the mother produced disturbed behavioural patterns such as autistic rocking, fear, aggression, withdrawal, apathy, and hyperactivity. And as these monkeys grew up, they had poor social interaction skills and were unable to mate. Harlow's experiments clearly demonstrate the infant's need for "contact comfort" and its effect on emotional development.

There have been a number of human studies of the results of contact comfort on a child's personality and development. Dr. Margaret Ribble studied the effects of infant care after birth. She was concerned with procedures used in hospitals that included separating the infant from the mother. In one case, infants were kept in a special sterile nursery for long periods of time, with little physical handling by either the nursing staff or the mother. Dr. Ribble reported that nearly a third of some 600 newborns in the study showed patterns of intense muscular tension. She noted that this tension was relieved when the baby was in close physical contact with the mother – sucking, or being rocked or cuddled. Dr. Ribble reported that infants who do not get such physical mothering may develop a condition called "marasmus," which includes such symptoms as poor muscle tone, a protruding belly, poor skin colour and – for some – liver congestion.

Positive changes in hospital procedure have resulted from such findings. In well-administered facilities, infants today are given immediately to their mothers and in some cases are kept in the same room.

According to some researchers, *physical contact between mother and child may be a specific inhibitor of distress for both of them.*

Another researcher, Dr. R.A. Spitz, studied the lack of mothering among foundling-home babies and noted a condition he called "anaclitic depression." Symptoms included loss of appetite, developmental retardation, lack of awareness of the environment, and sleeping problems. According to yet another researcher, Dr. Franck, infants initially need physical comfort in varying degrees, and such comfort is essential for their development. He further claims that denial of these early tactile experiences may affect their cognition, their ability to learn such skills as speech, and their capacity for physical tactile communication as adults.

PHYSICAL COMFORTING AND AUTISM

One of the severe childhood disturbances linked to the absence of physical comforting is infantile autism. Autistic children are characterized by an extreme degree of unresponsiveness to their total environment. They seem to live in a world of their own, completely engrossed in self-stimulatory behaviour such as rocking back and forth for hours, flapping their wrists, and – in some extreme cases – self-mutilation. This self-destructiveness often takes the form of biting themselves and severe head-banging. They display an obsession with sameness, and become very anxious in unfamiliar environments. Their speech is badly impaired and some autistic children are mute or have an echolaic speech pattern (repeating words spoken by others). To date, traditional psychotherapeutic methods have not been very successful. Behaviour therapy and reinforcement techniques have resulted in some dramatic but limited change, as has play therapy.

Professor Harvey Mandel and his associates, who investigated the causes and treatment of autism, maintain that one of the causes for this condition may be physical contact deprivation in infancy. They state: "the issue is that at the critical point of early infancy, the child did not receive a basic mothering experience through the medium of physical involvement."

From their clinical experience, Dr. Mandel's group discovered that some parents of autistic children were highly verbal and related to their infant verbally, but not physically, and that they deprived the infant of significant security experiences which come from physical mothering (cuddling, bathing, and feeding). They conclude that because the infant has a high need for physical sensory stimulation and is physically/emotionally deprived, he retreats within himself and is forced into self-stimulation to satisfy his basic needs.

He is in a sensory and emotional vacuum unable to do anything but wait for the special relationship he needs. This becomes increasingly difficult to find because (1) the physical mothering relationship becomes a less and less likely parental response with increasing chronological age; and (2) the deficits in developmental skill become almost insurmountable as the years go by. If the autistic child manages to reach chronological adulthood, he is probably indistinguishable from the severely retarded.

Other investigators have agreed with the Mandel group and have suggested that – because of rejection – the autistic child protects himself by creating an impregnable shield, behind which he satisfies his needs for sensory stimulation.

In their treatment program, based on their assumption that some forms of autism may be caused by physical sensory deprivation, Dr. Mandel and his colleagues have attempted to fulfil these needs. The therapist literally "feeds" the child sensory experiences (tickling, swinging, cuddling, and so forth). An entry from their casebook provides us with some appreciation for and understanding of these techniques:

> ...I gradually began to tickle him, hug him, swing him and with my physical support, let him use some of the gym equipment. Alan would now drop most of his rituals when I approached him and his body was generally more relaxed, but he would stiffen up if I left him.

> Alan now pushes the other children away from me and demands that I swing him.

> For the last month, he has been looking at people straight in the eye and has been coming up to complete strangers. He is also beginning to explore other rooms at the school and outdoors.

The therapists reported that after eight months of treatment, which included a substantial measure of physical contact, one child became more aware of his environment, lost some of his physical rigidity, and reacted positively when hugged. He initiated contact with people, began to make sounds, and generally seemed to thrive on physical comforting and activity.

Most consequences of physical-sensory deprivation are not as devastating as the autistic sickness treated by Dr. Mandel and his associates, but the consequences of such deprivation may range on a scale from minor personality and adjustment difficulties to severe psychological disturbances in childhood and adulthood. Investigations like the Mandel study give us important insights and direction.

Dr. James W. Prescott, a developmental neuropsychologist at the National Institute of Child Health and Human Development in the United States, reports that certain specific studies suggest that some kinds of sensory deprivation – including a lack of touching and rocking by the mother – could result in incomplete development of the neuronal systems during the formative period of brain growth. In short, the structure of the brain can be affected. Prescott's investigations disclosed a significant relationship between physical affection shown to human infants and rates of adult physical violence. "In one study of 49 primitive cultures, I found that when levels of infant affection are low, levels of violence are high; when physical affection is high, as among the Maori of New Zealand and the Balinese, violence is low ... the possible lesson for modern countries is clear. We seem to be suffering from a breakdown in affectional bonds – reflected in everything from rates of divorce to sexual crimes, alcoholism and drug abuse and without a proper environment for physical affection, a peaceful harmonious society may not be possible."

The work of Dr. John Bowlby, an eminent child psychiatrist, also clearly emphasizes the effects of the deprivation of maternal and paternal care on the physical, intellectual, emotional, and social development of the child, as well as the specific importance of nurturance in the "bonding" between mother and child. There are critical time periods in a child's development when this affectional, physical nurturance is necessary; if it is not there, the attachment or bonding does not take place.*

Physical contact is a reciprocal transaction between two people. For the child it is a significant act that conveys a message which says "I love you, I care for you, and I will take care of you." It is a warm blanket of emotional and physical security, of unrestrained acceptance. Deep emotions are also invoked in the parent by physical contact with the child. What do *you* feel when you hug your baby? When you kiss the soft face, or nuzzle the infant? There are no words to describe adequately those warm, tender, loving feelings. It's a special "high." All the pains of labour, and of difficult days and nights of care, are washed away by this delicious sensation: *two hugs for survival* – an apt prescription for the well-being of both child and parent.

ADULT NEEDS FOR PHYSICAL CONTACT

Sidney Jourard, one of the founders of the humanistic psychology

---

*A group of Harvard researchers have shown that children who receive physical affection especially from their fathers grow up better able to cope with stress and to adapt to new situations and people.

movement, studied physical contact in adulthood and its relationship to sound mental health. His findings suggest that many people suffer from a deprivation of physical contact during their adult lives. "I have seen happily married spouses touch one another dozens of times ... and miserably married persons whom I have seen in psychotherapy have often complained of too little physical contact."

Jourard refers to touching as an instinctual need and states that physical contact may indeed be a natural sedative and tranquilizer, free of the dangerous side effects of pharmaceutical compounds. It was his conviction that some people turn to drugs because they do not receive enough physical contact or caressing in their everyday lives. Jourard studied hospital care in the United States and was concerned about the absence of physical contact between the nurses and doctors and their patients. It was almost avoidance, predicated both on official hospital policy and on the "touch taboo" that has developed in our society. Nurses would dispense needed drugs but not the physical comfort or psychotherapeutic touch needed to speed the healing process.

When my mother was convalescing in a senior-citizen hospital following a serious hip operation, I would visit her every day. We would greet each other with a hug and kiss, and while we sat and talked she would hold my hand. It was a very special time of day for both of us. I could sense how much she seemed to need this physical closeness. She knew when to expect me and would sit by the elevator in her wheelchair, waiting.

Soon some of her new friends began to gather by the elevator, and over a period of time, I began to hold their hands or put my arm around their shoulders. It became a routine when I arrived and departed. There was such a hunger for contact, and such appreciation for a touch. The nursing staff and social workers seemed forever involved with pills and bingo cards, but they seldom had time for a gentle, friendly touch. Their busyness, their preoccupation with other matters, left no moments free for the very thing those in pain and distress needed most – physical affection.

TOUCH TABOOS

Dr. Jourard points out that there are individual variations in the need for physical contact, and that some individuals live with invisible fences around their bodies. These individuals feel safe within this fence and keep others at a "proper" physical distance. They panic if someone invades this private space.

I have worked with child-abuse victims who have built such fences and who cannot tolerate having anyone approach them with any physical affection. Many have been victimized and never develop normal interpersonal relationships. You can't get close to them. Many adults become annoyed and jump if touched on the shoulder during conversations or meetings.

Touch avoidance is not always the result of early rejection or physical abuse. We must also recognize that needs may vary from individual to individual. But much avoidance is learned in the home, partly because of the "touch taboo" that prevails in our culture. Still, if there is so much evidence of the importance of physical contact, why the *touch taboo*?

Touching is a language, and it can convey many messages, such as:

I like you
I love you
I care about you
I will take care of you
I feel badly for your sorrow
Congratulations
Thank you
Everything will be all right

It can also mean "I need some physical affection."

Hugging is regarded as acceptable at births, weddings, and funerals. Athletes hug and embrace to celebrate a touchdown, or home run, or any kind of victory. Politicians engage in baby kissing, embracing, and handshaking. If touching is such a significant act of goodwill, why the taboo?

One answer may be that touching can also convey a sexual message and a hidden agenda. There is a fear that what might be an innocent touch is really a sexual or lustful touch. Freud may have created or accelerated the taboo with his concept of the "Oedipal complex." There is a fear or concern that physical contact may have an incestuous or homosexual motive. These fears have influenced behaviour in our society. Fathers are careful in their physical contact with their daughters after the age of twelve, and many stop hugging their sons after the age of seven or eight. Instead we shake hands, because we think handshaking appears *more masculine* and less threatening.

If, as the evidence suggests, one needs two hugs for survival, and if physical contact is a specific inhibitor of distress in children and adults, what is the cost to society of this phobic touch taboo and of the invisible fences we build around ourselves? Is a change in our attitude possible?

POSITIVE CHANGES

I'm optimistic about the changes taking place in our society, and I think they are taking place for many reasons. Many people are presently undergoing psychotherapy whose defensiveness is being reduced, who are becoming more open, more in touch with their need for physical contact, and less bound by or concerned about the perceptions of others or about societal myths. We have also learned from the young, whose spontaneous embrace is part of their language of acceptance, support, and honesty. They are not as concerned about hidden agendas or as afraid of the commitments some people associate with a hug. The macho image is being challenged and changed, so that to have emotions, to *show* emotions by physical contact – be it a touch on the hand or shoulder, or an embrace – is not perceived as an act peculiar to the feminine domain but rather as basic human behaviour responding to basic human needs.

Such an act is reciprocal, because it affects the person who is hugged and the person who is hugging. It is contagious. It gives a message that cannot be matched by or articulated in any other language.

Finally, two hugs for survival is, of course, just a manner of speaking. The number – two – is merely suggestive. It really means: give your children lots of contact comfort, spontaneously and naturally. You will not spoil them if the comfort is genuinely given, without strings. And don't cut the practice off at any age. Effectiveness and enjoyment in parenting begin with such demonstrations of love, but such acts are not, of course, by themselves sufficient. There are many other important ways of saying "I love you."

But Love Is More than a Hug

Whenever I ask a group of parents about the skills they consider necessary to be an effective parent there is always someone who answers: "The basic skill is the ability to love. A child thrives and grows on love."

Whether or not love is a skill and whether or not it is sufficient depend on one's definition of love and on the motive for the loving. If one were to define parental love as Webster defines love, in terms of affection and fondness, it would *not* be enough. If the motive for loving, as we often see in our clinics, reflects personal needs, selfishness, low self-esteem, fear of the loss of the child's love, or compensation for an absence of love in marriage or for an unconscious dislike for the child, this love is negative and leads to immaturity and insecurity. Though children are sensitive to real love, because of their vulnerability they can also be smothered and spoiled with negative loving. As a captive audience, children may mimic and internalize the unwholesome motives of imperfect love.

THE HIT-AND-KISS PHENOMENON

A real scenario. It's been a crummy day for Linda! John has been away on a sales trip for three days and just called to say that he's sorry but it's going to take him another day to complete all his calls. Jamie and Jill have been up for nights with fever and chicken pox. Skipper got into a fight with another dog and needed ten stitches to repair his ear. The bank called about a "little" overdraft. But the straw that broke Linda's fragile balance was John's mother who phoned to say, "John is working too hard and should try to get away fishing." Wham! Jamie got it, and Jill hid from the screaming and hitting. Even Skipper got his butt kicked out the door.

Following the storm and the wreckage Linda just sat and cried and then began to treat the physically and emotionally wounded with a large dose of loving, hugging, and kissing. And this was her pattern: "Let Mommy make it all better with a kiss." It may soothe for a moment but there are scars and confusion that are not erased. By itself this type of love is not enough. Children can figure out that punishment follows a misdemeanour but love following punishment, especially when there is innocence, is a confused message. What do they learn from this "schizy" sequence of behaviour? "Love is what you get or what you use after you hit someone smaller – it's how Mommy and Daddy say I'm sorry." What a sad lesson! There must be more to parental love.

THE INGREDIENTS OF PARENTAL LOVE

Various factors or ingredients of parental love are necessary for the healthy emotional growth of children. Dorothy Corkville Briggs, in an excellent book titled *Your Child's Self-Esteem,* outlines the seven active ingredients of parents' nurturing love for their children. According to Dr. Briggs, these include *genuine encounters*, which deal with undivided attention to the child, plus six others she categorizes under *psychological safety*. The six are: safety of trust, safety of parental non-judgement, safety of being cherished, safety of owning feelings, safety of empathy, and safety of being allowed to be unique. As Dr. Briggs explains, "When these ingredients are then combined in an atmosphere of warm affection and physical contact, a child feels loved, secure, and can grow emotionally, physically, and intellectually and becomes capable of giving this nurturing love to others."

FROMM'S CONDITIONAL AND UNCONDITIONAL LOVE

For Erich Fromm, the renowned psychoanalyst, loving is an act that is more than mere sentiment. In his view, love requires understanding, *practice*, concentration, maturity, self-knowledge, faith, courage, and self-discipline.

In his book *The Art of Loving*, Dr. Fromm distinguishes between "unconditional love," which he calls mother love, and "conditional love," which he calls father love, and points out the positive and negative aspects of these two types of love. The use of "mother" in "mother love" and "father" in "father love" are merely figures of speech, since fathers are capable of "mother love" and mothers are capable of "father love." In fact, both kinds of love can exist in any parent.

Unconditional love, which is the first love a child experiences, is a natural, "instinctive" love that does not have to be earned, deserved, or acquired. It is just *there*. "I am loved because I am." This love is unconditional; it provides warmth and security. That's the positive side of unconditional love. The negative side is that such love *cannot* be acquired, controlled, or created. If a mother does not have this euphoric feeling, it does not develop. To be loved unconditionally is a deep longing in most human beings.

Conditional love, which Fromm calls "father love," is *earned* love. It is earned when a child fulfils his father's expectations, when he carries out his duties, and when he becomes like his father. The negative aspect of fatherly love is that it is given only for obedience. When a child is disobedient, this fatherly love is withdrawn. But its positive aspect emphasizes that, since love is conditional, *you* are in control, and you can *acquire* this love merely by fulfilling father's expectations.

For healthy growth, a child needs both loves. Mother love gives him security. After the age of six, "father love" prepares and guides and teaches him to cope with the inevitable problems he will face. "Father love" is patient and tolerant and allows for growth of independence.

The mature parent, according to Fromm, is a synthesis of conditional and unconditional love. When this synthesis fails to develop in the parent, neurosis may result in the child. Neurosis sets in when there is only mother love, and father love is absent. If mother is over-indulgent and domineering, and if father is weak and uninvolved in the caretaking, the child remains fixated at an early stage of development. He remains dependent and helpless and lacks the ability ever to direct his own life. Another one-sided development described by Fromm results from the absence of unconditional love and the dispensing of conditional love alone. A child thus treated becomes obsessed with law, order, and authority and is incapable of receiving or giving unconditional love.

Mother love is the basis for all else that follows. Fromm uses biblical symbolism to compare mother love to the promised land, which flows with milk and honey. He uses milk as the symbol of affirmation and care, and honey as the symbol of the sweetness of life and love for life. Most mothers can supply the milk, but only a few are capable of bestowing honey. When a mother is a truly happy person, her joy becomes contagious, and the child develops a personality that demonstrates joy in being alive.

Fromm also feels that a mother's love must include the desire for her children's eventual independence and the ability to survive the separation. A mother who is secure in her own existence, and whose love is unconditional, weathers such changes and welcomes the shift from dependence to independence.

This conception of the art of loving is reality-based, acknowledging and encouraging our natural feelings of love without strings, together with a love based on the fulfilment of expectations and duties in an environment of patience and support. For too many, love is an either/or phenomenon. Fromm helps us to understand that mature love is a synthesis of conditional and unconditional love.

My only concern with Dr. Fromm's position is his support of the withdrawal of love as a reprimand for disobedience. This pulls the rug from under the child and endangers his emotional security. A parent can openly disapprove of a specific negative behaviour and withdraw a privilege as a sanction. The privilege might be the child's allowance, or permission to watch TV, or use of the family car. But being loved should not be classified as a privilege along with permission to watch a favourite program or to receive spending money every Friday.

LOVE: AN ATTITUDE WITH THREE BASIC ELEMENTS

Historically, children have been considered the property of their parents. The right of parents to abuse, neglect, scream at, or spank their offspring has long been viewed as a private, unquestioned right. It has taken many years for any Declaration of Children's Rights to be recognized.

Children are not party to your decision that they be brought into this world. But once they arrive, they have a fundamental right to the expectation that they are entering a nurturing environment whose essence is positive and loving. This loving attitude is demonstrated to the child through three basic elements of love: (1) *feeling*, (2) *belief*, and (3) *action*.

The *feeling* is that expressed in Fromm's concept of unconditional love: "I am loved because I am." It is not a feeling of love to be acquired or deserved; the feeling exists because "I have been created by my parents."

Unconditional love – and not a "wait until I see what you're like" love – may be the child's first right, but it is not by itself sufficient. The second element of a loving attitude is a *belief*, and this is the child's second right. Parental belief includes faith in the child's potential and uniqueness and confidence in themselves to become competent parents. It is a belief that the role parents had in the child's creation does not end at birth. Instead, the act of creation continues through loving, inspiring, and teaching our children, and by encouraging the development of all the potential energy and resources our children possess.

Love is made complete only when feeling and belief are translated into *action*. A child has the right to action by the parent. The feeling of love may be a source of energy; the belief gives love value and direction. But action is the ultimate expression of love. Energy, direction, and expression of love are the three basic rights of a child, and all must be present if there is to be healthy growth and development.

It is not enough merely to have feelings of love, or simply to express those feelings with a hug. It is not enough to simply have faith, since this vulnerable organism – the child – will not make it in this world unless his parents seek information on child-rearing, come to understand it, learn the needed skills and strategies, and remain continuously involved in the child-rearing process from infancy to adulthood. What is continuous, loving involvement? It starts with the satisfaction of a child's basic needs – feeding, bathing, changing, hugging, and gentling. It continues with singing, reading, playing, and teaching. It includes exploration and testing in an atmosphere where failure is acceptable. Then, as the child grows, there is discussion, listening, explanation, focused attention, the sharing of thoughts, plans, experiences, and expectations, and the laying down of rules and duties in the family and society.

These are some of the ways in which love for a child can be expressed. But it is not enough merely to commit one's self to be involved. Parenting is a very special profession. In no other profession is one so emotionally and intimately involved, and in no other profession is there such a wide variety of skills to be mastered. For this most complicated of all professions, parents are the least trained and worst prepared, as the incidence of failure dramatically testifies. As noted earlier, 41 per cent of the parents we questioned in a recent survey reported that parenting had been a frustrating, negative experience. Many of them said they would not have children if they could live their lives over again. This is a sad commentary on the status of parenthood in our society.

Still, examination of the 22 per cent who qualified parenting as "fulfilling" gives us some direction. Much of what we learned should have been obvious. The major difference between the two groups lies not in their *feelings* of love for their children, but in their *belief in* and *expression of* love. They never waited to say "I love you." Many parents have regretted that they waited too long before they verbalized their feelings of affection, and their children in turn never learned to openly and easily express their "I love you." A child's best mode of learning is by modelling and imitation. What they see and what they hear is often what they do.

FOUR

A One-to-One Relationship:

A Strategy for Effective Communication

One important way I show my love is to show myself...my past, my hopes, my disappointment, my excitement, my anger, my sadness, my tenderness, my body, my time, my secrets, my skills, my energy, my reactions to the world...it is an opening process that gradually gives another person the gifts I have to give.

— JOHN WOOD

"There is something special and sacred about a relationship between two people that is lost when there are three or four or more. A one-to-one relationship cements, heals, resolves, and builds...it feels good."

If I were limited to only one suggestion for success in parenting, it would be: *"Develop a one-to-one relationship with your children."* Clinical and experimental research, and my own personal experiences as a parent, convince me that such a relationship is the most powerful foundation for emotional, intellectual, and social growth, and for the fulfilment of both parent and child.

Success in parenting should be measured not only in terms of "child growth" but also in terms of "parent growth." If the growing years have been enjoyable ones for both parent and offspring, and if the relationship continues strong and pleasurable long after the children have left home, it is probable that a close one-to-one association has existed in the family from the beginning.

A close one-to-one relationship between parent and child is perhaps the most basic and productive of all human relationships. The emotional bonds that develop help both parent and child to cope with the inevitable traumas of growth. A closeness of hearts and of minds is nurtured that makes parenting a fulfilling adventure and a successful experience.

From our survey and our many interviews with parents, one very significant factor kept being emphasized. "Much of our success as parents comes from the fact that we really know our children and they know us because we spend a lot of time with them individually. It's easy to communicate with them on a one-to-one basis."

Question 17:
Do you spend time together with your child on a one-to-one basis?

Results:
1. Of the 22 per cent who thought of parenting as a "fulfilling and enjoyable" experience, 77 per cent reported having one-to-one relationships with their children.

2. Of the 37 per cent who reported they found parenting "moderately fulfilling and sometimes enjoyable," only 30 per cent had such relationships with their youngsters.

3. Of the 41 per cent who regarded parenting as "frustrating, negative, and not enjoyable," only 18 per cent indicated they had established one-to-one relationships with their children.

These results clearly establish a significant association between the one-to-one relationship and success in parenting. Although many factors determine your success as a parent, perhaps the most important is the closeness of your relationship with your children. Parents who enjoy their roles and who seem to be good at parenting have set aside special time to be with their children on a one-to-one basis. They appear to have taken this initiative beginning very early in the child's life and to have continued it up through adolescence and beyond. The one-to-one association has extended to all kinds of human activity, in a variety of situations and settings.

Parents who chronically have problems with their children – especially in the adolescent years – seldom have developed a closeness with their children. Their reasons may range from "it never occurred to me" to "I just didn't have the time." For most of these parents, home is a battleground rather than a haven. For them, child-rearing is one continuing crisis, a period of trauma when adolescents may ask "when do I get out?" and parents respond "I can't wait." In such families, parents and children are like ships passing in the night, with built-in radar devices to avoid all contact. Each family member pursues his or her own course, a voyage of the uninvolved, with contact occurring, if ever, purely by chance.

This certainly doesn't portray every family all of the time, but the high frequency of such situations is of concern. It fairly portrays many of the 41 per cent who report parenting as frustrating and negative. Many factors contribute to the unhappy family described: parents' lack of understanding of child development; lack of parenting skills; negative attitude towards parenting. The problems may be compounded by both parents working and having limited time available for their children. Some parents have abdicated responsibility to professionals and other agents for child-rearing and training – teachers, physicians, psychologists, tutors, or Children's Aid Societies. With a high rate of separations and divorce in our society, the pressure of a splitting or severed relationship between the parents is also a factor. Ambivalent parental attitudes also confuse and destroy relationships, e.g., an attitude that vascillates from a "I must do my own thing" to "our family must have total togetherness." Finally, the absence of a meaningful one-to-one relationship between the parents themselves and between the parents and their children leads to a deteriorating family situation, since they do not have relationships to help them weather the storms and turbulence of growing.

What Is a One-to-One Relationship?

Is a "one-to-one" merely two people coming together to talk, eat, play tennis, argue – or whatever? Not really. In the sense used in this book, a one-to-one relationship is something very special, something that evolves from a parent's caring and a child's responding. Such a relationship is delicate and fragile, nurtured by time and involvement, and may serve many basic needs, including:

- the instinctual need for physical comfort
- the need to belong
- the need for feedback
- the need for cheering up
- the need for help in goal achievement
- the need for a model to emulate
- the need to play
- the need for a close friend

A true "one-to-one" creates a special climate in which – because we care – we listen carefully to another's accounts of successes or failures, dreams or anxieties, fears, frustrations, and fantasies. We listen, for a moment in time, without sitting as judge or jury, and with sensitive regard for the other's self-esteem.

In an ideal one-to-one relationship children will share their inner-most thoughts and experiences without reservation. These are magical moments when children or parents may disclose ambivalent feelings toward one another, of like and dislike, of approach and avoidance...moments when sharing, understanding, and problem-solving take precedence over damning or apologizing or the saving up of information to be used as future ammunition.

When a parent discloses his innermost feelings to a child, or shares his thoughts, feelings, and experiences, he is making a powerful statement to that youngster. He is saying, in substance: "I trust you. I respect your judgement and your confidence. I need your love and your support." Such a statement gives an enormous assist to the development of a young child's or an adolescent's self-concept. Such a child grows up without facing the "feet of clay" disillusionment which follows when the myth of the all-powerful, all-knowing, invincible parent is at last shattered or eroded. This trauma often happens in adolescence, when cracks begin to appear in the shining parental armour.

A parent who has sensitively pursued a one-to-one relationship with his child or children has, in the process, let his offspring know that he, the parent, can be wrong, can hurt, can cry, can fear, can sometimes be confused, can at times have ambivalent feelings, and can dream. This, for the parent, leads to a more honest existence and allows him to concentrate on coping with the stresses and realities of everyday life rather than preoccupying himself with preserving an idealized but strictly cosmetic image. This parental disclosure acts as a model for the child and gives the child licence to share her or his innermost feelings, thoughts, and actions. For the child, such an environment encourages growth away from preoccupation with her or his own selfish world and toward greater understanding of and consideration for others.

But perhaps the most important consequence, the most dramatic payoff to come from an active one-to-one relationship, lies in the ways in which such a relationship can help both parents and youngsters to face up to, and overcome, the hurdles and agonies of that most critical period of all: adolescence, the so-called age of emancipation and rebellion.

The Age of Emancipation and Rebellion

The normal growing process includes moving from a stage of dependency to a stage of independence, and then to the final and most mature stage: a blend of independence and interdependency (see Figure 4). Interdependency is being dependent on someone and having someone dependent on you. Complete independence is, of course, a myth since every human being has so many needs that can be fulfilled only by others: family, friends, societal groups, the mailman, the policeman, the farmer, physicians – and even the weather.

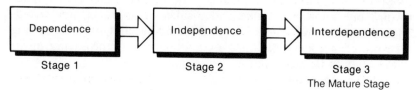

Figure 4. The Growth to Interdependence

The transition from dependency to independence awakens feelings in the adolescent of bewilderment, turmoil, frustration, fright, impatience, anger, and resentment. For many, these feelings heat up and boil over, causing them to strike out at others or inward toward themselves, or to flee or fight. On their part, the parents of adolescents sometimes react with feelings of anxiety, anger, frustration, concern, or bewilderment, and may at this time ask themselves "Where did I go wrong?"

This is a momentous period for many adolescents, during which the no-longer child but not-yet adult is called upon to

- adjust to new physical and hormonal changes;
- develop a sense of self-identity;
- adopt adult roles;
- accept new responsibilities and new rules of conduct;
- explore sexuality;
- decide on vocational objectives;
- adjust to a new balance of power and decision-making in the family;
- seek peer acceptance; and
- face the loss of security that had come automatically with dependency.

Some of the psychological changes that occur in adolescence are listed by Professor Hurlock, including:

- a desire for isolation and privacy;
- heightened emotionality caused by hormonal changes, resulting in sudden outbursts of anger, impatience, a tendency to cry easily;
- excessive modesty;
- lack of co-ordination due to an inability to adjust quickly to rapidly changing body size;
- insecurity which becomes manifest as decreased self-confidence; and
- confusion arising from periods of mature behaviour followed by immature behaviour – "flip-flop" feelings and "flip-flop" behaviour.

The consequences of these changes include such acting-out behaviour as use of drugs or alcohol, premarital sex, flight from home, early marriages, pregnancies, and suicides. Statistics establish clearly that such consequences are not isolated incidents, that millions of adolescents experience one or more of the above behaviour patterns as consequences of their stress and turmoil. These are the most visible and dramatic consequences. Others include the breakdown of rational communications at home, emotional over-reactions, and the break-up of relationships.

It is a difficult time – it is an *inevitable* time. Yet this period does not have to terminate with dire consequences. It is a time in a young person's life requiring from parents high levels of understanding, patience, love, support, communication, and, most of all, a long prior history of one-to-one relationships. Ideally the history starts in infancy, then grows and matures through early childhood, middle childhood, and adolescence. What should develop, in these twelve to fourteen years, is a *habit* deeply engrained in both parent and child of enjoying one another, of talking and listening to one another, of sharing confidences and failures, successes and fantasies, of risking intimate disclosures without fear of reprimand, of testing new skills and declaring new needs and new feelings. Conflicts are not in themselves bad. How a conflict is resolved is the critical learning.

By the time the age of emancipation and rebellion arrives, the habit is so deeply engrained that trust, deep affection, and easy communication exist between parent and child. This firm relationship can then be called upon to help both parties to ride out the crisis. How serious is this crisis? Recently on CBS television it was reported that over *one million children* have run away from home and that many are in serious trouble. They are involved in drugs, alcohol, prostitution, porno films, and crime. Most do not run away from an environment that has been warm, open, empathetic, and enjoyable. Many of these runaways were going through the turbulence of adolescence in a "regime" where there is no habit or history of one-to-one communication, where everyone is shouting, reprimanding, or denying, but where no one is listening to the intensity of needs, frustration, or anger. When there is no long-standing, warm, trusting relationship, parents, in their dilemma, try to control, restrict, invoke, and punish, and in the process they generally create more heat than light in the situation. The result is a bust-out, a break-up, a runaway.

Parents who seek counselling during this difficult period sometimes ask: "If we have not developed a one-to-one relationship before this difficult age of rebellion, is it too late?" Fortunately, the answer is "no." It is not too late, but it is more difficult. Obviously it is easier to develop such a relationship beginning in infancy and through early childhood, when there is plenty of time to learn and develop together. However, it is possible to develop a one-to-one at any age and stage.

Elements of a One-to-One Relationship

Certain basic elements in a sound one-to-one must be there before such a relationship will grow. These are understanding, acceptance, trust, empathy, open communication, time, and motivation.

MOTIVATION

Very little learning takes place without motivation; it is the energizer and mobilizer, and it gives direction to your behaviour. The equation for successful performance in all spheres is: Motivation x Instruction x Practice = Successful Performance. There has to be a strong motivation to *want* to be with and to be part of the excitement of your child's growing up physically, emotionally, intellectually, and socially. The parents must want to maximize the child's potential, to enjoy not only the attainment of goals but the process of the growth. The motivation to want to learn the parenting skills to facilitate this growth and a willingness to accept the bumps of growing must also be present.

TIME

Time is an important ingredient in the building of a one-to-one relationship. Too many parents cite "lack of time" as an excuse for their failure to forge such relationships. Let's face it: having time is a matter of reshuffling priorities. What is really more important – a church meeting, or sharing some precious moments with your child? Time with children should be a parent's number one priority, and schedules should be adjusted accordingly.

It is critical that parents recognize one central fact: strong, meaningful relationships can be developed only with time; there is no such thing as an "instant" one-to-one. A parent who is preoccupied with "how long should it take?" would be well-advised to let the process take as long as necessary and should bear in mind, as well, that the quality of time spent is the more significant factor.

THE LEARNING-HOPE CURVE

Is a one-to-one relationship natural or learned? I think it is both. Therefore, if it doesn't feel entirely natural at first, don't stop trying; you can learn to enjoy a one-to-one. For most of us, the learning process passes through the stages depicted in Figure 5.

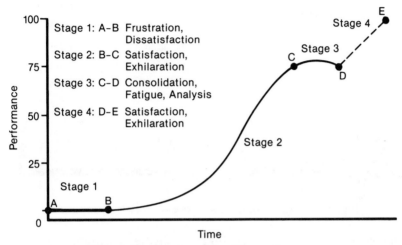

Figure 5. The Learning-Hope Curve

All learning follows a similar process, whether it is learning to play tennis or the guitar, becoming a mechanic or a surgeon, or learning the elements of a one-to-one relationship. At least four stages are involved. The beginning, Stage 1, may be marked by awkwardness, discomfort, and dissatisfaction with the trial and error progress: "Will it *ever* come?" Stage 2, a period of comfort and satisfactions, may arrive suddenly: "It's happened...it's getting better and better...I really feel comfortable when I'm with that kid." Stage 3 follows, when there is consolidation, a maturing. This is an easy period, which can be a prelude to the final level, Stage 4, when both parties will say, "I enjoy our times together and look forward to them."

Parents who understand the entire learning process are better able to cope with Stage 1, a period of discomfort and trial and error, knowing that a period of comfort (Stage 2) will eventually come, followed by more improvements in Stages 3 and 4. Although this is a predictable process, many parents quit at Stage 1 and never taste the success.

SHARING YOURSELF: AN INVITATION

One of the most powerful ingredients in the development of a one-to-one relationship is the disclosure of one's real self to a child. Sharing some intimate facet of yourself often gives the child licence to share himself

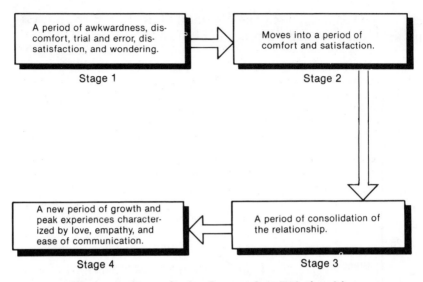

Figure 6. Stages in the One-to-One Relationship

with you. This involvement on your part – the free disclosure of details about your childhood, your dreams, your failures and successes, your worries, the true picture of your everyday world – changes a one-way communication system characterized by questioning, reprimanding, and ordering to a two-way relationship marked by trust, understanding, caring, and excitement.

Many parents are amazed to find how little their children know about their past or their present, and how much they want to know. My children were forever asking their grandmother what I was like when I was a little boy and delighted in her accounts – how I accidentally burned down the garage, about my first girl friend, about how she felt when she put me on a train, alone, to visit Aunt Hilda in Cleveland (and I got off at the wrong station!).

A parent's past and present are sometimes regarded as private preserves, restricted and off limits. Yet we, as parents, want and expect to know everything about our children's lives: where they have been, with whom, and what they did to the finest detail. Do we keep such information from our children because we fear we will damage our image? Or do we assume that our youngsters aren't old enough to understand, or that they really don't care?

Parents with whom we have consulted reveal that, when they begin to share themselves – especially if the sharing involves disclosure of some difficult experience from their past or present – a remarkable change takes place in the parent-child relationship. For the first time, the child may demonstrate openly his feelings of care and concern about his parent.

One father had experienced problems with his employer. The employer had verbally abused him, yelling at him and embarrassing him in front of fellow employees. He told his thirteen-year-old daughter about this experience, explaining how it affected his work and his self-image. With tears in her eyes, his daughter began to hug her father, and her tears and her concern brought tears to the father's eyes. His daughter had never seen her father cry and had never shared his hurts. She expressed her anger with her father's boss and said she wanted to do something terrible to him for hurting her father.

This experience established a bond with his daughter that the father had never felt before, and it changed their entire relationship. It was a good feeling, this closeness. They began to talk seriously with one another, and for the first time his daughter opened up to share her problems and her fears. She didn't need a therapist; she had a father who listened, who could be hurt just as she could, who cared, and who helped her to solve her problems.

Until this one-to-one relationship was established, this had been a family of loners – ships passing in the night. What contact there was consisted of charges and counter-charges, loud noises but little real listening. Even the husband-wife relationship was progressively deteriorating on the family battleground. The building of a strong father-daughter relationship helped to repair the damage.

THE VALUE OF EMPATHY

Empathy is a precious ability. It means that when your child shares confidences with you, his innermost feelings, his rational and irrational thoughts, his problems or his experiences, you listen carefully and for a moment in time you are not *judge* or *jury*, but you are trying to *understand* and *experience* the child's feelings. You begin to feel what it must be like to be the child; you try to understand the child's alternatives and demonstrate a high degree of caring, of acceptance, of positive regard; you seek to preserve his own self-esteem. When this happens you can become an agent of support, of help and problem-solving. This helps to develop a sound communication network for present and future that can overcome many of the causes of stress in growing up for a parent or for a child.

Instead of angry parental monologues of reprimand, insult, and instruction and instead of a child or adolescent's monologue of denial or defensiveness, there develops a dialogue that is based on listening, accepting, and experiencing what the other person is feeling. The preoccupation moves from the judgement and assessment of behaviour as good or bad to a total preoccupation with the solution to a problem. No energy is wasted on the protection of self-esteem and no years are lost from what could have been a special relationship.

A BAD SCENARIO

DAD: Why are you up so late?

DORA: I've got two exams tomorrow – biology and history. That makes six exams this week. I'm so tired…I know I'm going to fail. I just didn't schedule my time right.

DAD: I told you to begin studying earlier in the year. You never learn.

DORA: Oh, leave me alone! And close my door!

With his preaching and his reprimand, Dad achieved nothing here. He succeeded only in making Dora more anxious and less able to finish her studying, and drove the wedge between them even deeper.

A GOOD SCENARIO

DAD: Why are you up so late?

DORA: I've got two exams tomorrow – biology and history. That makes six exams this week. I'm so tired…I know I'm going to fail. I just didn't schedule my time right.

DAD: Six exams in one week is a heavy load, even though you have been working hard all year. You must be exhausted. Let me bring you a glass of orange juice.

DORA: With a glass of juice, and a hug from you, I think I'll make it!

Here, Dad was being empathetic. He could sense her tiredness and her anxiety, and he let his daughter know that he understood her feelings. It was not his agreement with her, but his understanding, that helped.
Here is another scenario, drawn from life.

A NEGATIVE SCENARIO

Dad is waiting in the family car to take Michael, age ten, to hockey practice. As Michael comes out the front door, Dad shouts:

DAD: Move it, Michael! You're always late. I hate sitting and waiting for you after a long day at work.

MICHAEL: I couldn't find my knee pads or my helmet.

DAD: You can never find anything. You're such a loser. Did you return those overdue books to the library and pay the fine?

MICHAEL: Yup.

DAD: Listen, when we get to the arena, please put your own skates on. I'm embarrassed to have to do up your laces. Your sweater is on backwards!

MICHAEL: (to himself) *What a bug! The only reason I'm playing hockey is because he makes me... I wish he'd let me take the bus!*

Dad may well have been tired from his hard day at the office and then having to fight traffic on the way home. But this was no justification for putting Michael down and shattering his self-esteem. The only possible result of Dad's antagonism and Michael's defensiveness will be a rift and mutual avoidance.

A POSITIVE SCENARIO

Dad is waiting in the family car to take Michael, age ten, to hockey practice. As Michael comes out the front door, Dad shouts:

DAD: Hi, Mike! I picked up Bobby Orr's book on hockey for you. It's really got some great tips on passing.

MICHAEL: That's terrific. I'm never where the puck is, and I could use some help.

DAD: Today was a hard day at work, and I'm really dragging. But I get a kick out of going to practice with you. Maybe we can have a little workout on the ice before next week's game – if you'll promise to take it easy on the old man!

MICHAEL: You can still skate rings around me, Dad. Do you think I'll make the team? I sure want to.

DAD: Well, if you don't, it won't be for lack of trying.

MICHAEL: (after a long silence) Dad... what was your father like? Did he play hockey?

DAD: My dad died when I was only four years old. I sure missed having a father. I used to pretend I had a father and tried to imagine what he was like and what we would do together. Sometimes I would pretend that my friend Herbie's father was my dad. Once he took Herbie and me to a father-and-son Boy Scout banquet – that was really something. When they introduced all the fathers and their sons, Herbie's dad grabbed my hand and Herbie's, and we all stood up. That was special!

In this one-to-one scenario, drawn from real life, father and son shared and enjoyed each other; they really cared. This is the kind of interpersonal climate that generates emotional security, self-esteem, and lasting companionship.

TOGETHERNESS

In counselling parents, I have found that there often is a conflict between their concept of "family togetherness" and my recommendations for one-to-one relationships. Why don't you go out alone with your son or daughter? Go for a walk or a movie. Take your son to your office to share your everyday world with him. Try this once or twice a week for a month. It gets easier and better with time. I have felt, at times, that these suggestions have violated their time-honoured definition of togetherness, which has customarily been viewed as something involving the entire family. Under this definition, there was – in their minds – no room for alternatives.

In reality, the one-to-one relationship *complements* family togetherness; it is proposed not as an alternative, but as a support. The benefits and joys that can come from family togetherness are well-documented, and the experiences gained can serve as models for our children to follow when they become parents. Family trips, sing-songs, ball games, barbecues, discussions, arguments: all are opportunities for learning to share, to adjust, to develop sensitivity, to enjoy family life. However, family togetherness can be carried to extremes, degenerating into a ritual or into an inflexibility which rejects any change. Or a homogeneity that submerges the individual character of the relationships between each pair of individuals. Under these circumstances, the results of togetherness can be negative. The following interview with a father (based on an actual case history) demonstrates how this may work, and it is not an atypical example:

What kinds of things do you do together, as a family?
Well, we eat together, watch TV together, take vacations together, read the paper together, go to the circus, the restaurants, to church – just about everything together. We really are a together family. I think it's important.

But do you enjoy it – this togetherness?
Most of the time. Sometimes it's a hassle…too many quarrels, too many different needs and moods. When we take a week's vacation together at the lake cottage, it takes us two weeks to recover at home.

If you had a choice, would you choose togetherness all the time?
NO!!!

If your wife and kids had a choice, would they prefer this "always togetherness"?
I don't think so.

Do you ever take one of your kids someplace, alone? Just the two of you?
I have done this, but rarely, because I don't have the time for both family outings and twosomes. Also, the other kids would get jealous and create a fuss.

Would you enjoy being with just one of your kids at a time?

I don't know what we would talk about, or do. It might be easier with my son. As for my daughters, we don't really have too much in common – there are such differences in age, language, and interests. It isn't as if I don't talk to them already, one-to-one. I always ask them how school is going, or what's new. And we discuss such things as their allowances....

How are things going at home?

Lots of hassles and shouting. It started with the "terrible twos" and continued through the "frightful fours," and every age and stage seems more difficult. I'm not sure my wife and I really have the patience, or the proper temperament, to be parents. I love my kids, but I'll be happy when they've gone. Right now we have a communication breakdown – everyone talks or yells, but no one listens. The kids certainly don't understand me, and I feel at times as if they don't even like me very much!

As I meet with parents during office visits, in clinics, and in workshops, "communication breakdown" is a theme constantly replayed: "I just don't have the time," or "We just don't understand one another," or "I'll be glad when they grow up and leave!" It's a sad theme, a tragic drama of unfulfilled expectations. Perhaps saddest of all is the waste – the waste, by two or more human beings, of the excitement of shared experience, and of the opportunity to forge a closeness which could enrich the lives of all concerned. In my meetings with these troubled families, I have noted that one common ingredient is missing in them all: none have developed close one-to-one relationships between parents and children.

In parenting workshops conducted over the past decade, I have used the following experiment to illustrate the value of the one-to-one relationship. I request a mother, a father, and one of their children to participate and ask each to enter a separate room near the common meeting room. These three separate rooms are linked by telephones. The three family members are given the simplest of tasks – for example, to decide what to have for dinner – and are asked to discuss the various possibilities and to arrive at a mutually satisfying decision. Their conversations are entirely by phone. This three-way conversation is piped into the room where the other workshop participants can overhear the results.

As the three try to arrive at a decision on what to have for dinner, the result is usually a mild form of chaos. While the adults pour out suggestions, the child usually zeroes in on pizza or lobbies for a visit to McDonald's. Predictably, there is little consensus. The "simple" task to which they have been assigned obviously turns out to be less than simple.

Voices are raised in frustration, heart rates go up, and there are desperate pleas for consideration so that one person can hear the other. Two people usually are talking at once. Finally, the most dominant personality takes over the conversation, which, it turns out, is no conversation at all. The child is usually the first to drop out, with occasional interruptions that are his or her way of saying: "If anyone is still listening, I'm still here."

I usually give the trio about five to ten minutes of this and break in just as the decibel level hits the eardrum discomfort zone. But by then the point has been made: human communication, to be effective, requires the following of certain ground rules. One of these is that one person should speak at a time, while the others listen. When more than two people are involved, someone in the group should "direct traffic." Otherwise, it is difficult to distinguish who is the "talker" and who the "listener." There is little real conversation, and a great deal of confusion and frustration.

After it is clear that not much is being achieved in this three-way telephone setup, I ask one of the adults to hang up and give the remaining two several minutes more to decide on what's for dinner. It's not surprising to hear great sighs of relief when the "survivors" realize they are "alone at last." Within seconds, the child is making more co-operative suggestions, and the parent is listening and responding.

The discussion that this experiment inspires in the workshop is so lively that I have come to realize it touches something critical in each of us. The struggle to be heard in a family discussion can be intense. Attempts by the younger, less articulate members to express their feelings or positions often become submerged as the "older, bigger, wiser" members of the family dominate the scene. However, if one-to-one relationships already have been established, there usually is better communication between and among all in such group discussions.

Each of us has a compelling need to be somehow "special," to feel unique, to be the centre of attention. In families, even if there is but one child, there is always competition, a kind of jockeying for position. We are all accustomed to this; it is natural. This does not mean, however, that there should not be moments, hours, or even days in which we are treated to the luxury of being alone with another member of the family. Some husbands and wives see the value of being away from the rest of the family and will spend evenings alone together and take vacations that do not include the children. But for many parents I have spoken with, the idea of developing a one-to-one relationship with a child had never occurred to them. True, the child's world may be different from the adult's, and it is a real challenge for each to enter into the other's world and be relaxed there, but the joy of mutual discovery, the closeness and warmth, make even rough attempts worthwhile.

We all remember happy times of family togetherness, but for most of us the "very special times" were those when it was just Mom and I, or Dad and I, on a fishing trip, in a restaurant, or during the night being cuddled for an ache or fever. These special times must not be left to chance. They should form part of a conscious, practised lifestyle. Innumerable parents have reported that, of all the "expert" recommendations they have heard, the most helpful and productive was "get to know your children, and let them get to know you, by spending time together – just the two of you."

And it gets better with time. Parents have reported that the technique has helped their children and themselves over many a difficult hurdle and has left them both with countless treasured memories. As one father remarked, with deep emotion: "This kid is now one of my best friends. Sometimes when we're together, we don't even have to talk. We just feel real good being together."

Early in my career as a child psychologist, I often recommended this idea of one-to-one relationships to new parents or parents with serious child-rearing problems. I made the recommendation, in those early times, not so much as a strategy based on scientific investigation, but rather because I had seen how effective and meaningful my own one-to-one experiences with my three daughters had been. I believe I know each of them really well, and they know me, as a father and as a special friend. Each one-to-one relationship was, and continues to be, unique and different. Yet we have all, individually and collectively, shared so much. My children are all mature adults now, in homes of their own, but geography is all that separates us. We are joined forever in mind and heart and share a good history that keeps us close.

Research and clinical evidence now substantiate this personal experience and philosophy of the value and desirability of such close one-to-one relationships as those our family built naturally many years ago.

One-to-One Relationships between Husband and Wife

Though the focus of this chapter has been the importance and the development of one-to-one relationships between parents and their children, it assumed that the basis for all family relationships is the husband-wife relationship. The intactness and style of the one-to-one relationship between husband and wife are certainly the model for all other one-to-ones in the family. A child's best mode of learning is by imitation: he mimics everything we do to our delight and to our chagrin. How Mom and Dad relate to each other, listen to each other, share with each other, care for each other, love, laugh and play together, argue, resolve, and spend one-to-one times together, sets the standard and the style in the family. It is and *must* be nurtured as the primary relationship.

It is there before the children arrive and must grow during the child-rearing years and endure and be enjoyed after the children depart.

Too many parents "park" their one-to-one relationship because of the supposed demands of the children. This is a misjudgement and can be fatal to their relationship and their relationships with their children. A relationship can rust out from non-use and may not be able to be repaired after fifteen or twenty years of parking. When parents tell me they have no time for themselves, that they are too tired from the burdens of child-rearing to enjoy each other sexually, emotionally, or intellectually, or can never take a holiday alone because of their belief in family togetherness, I suggest they "reshuffle" their priorities or they will suffer the consequences of alienation and of drift.

A problem with a child's behaviour usually motivates a parent to seek psychological help. After one or two interviews, the agenda often changes from "What's wrong with my child?" to "There are serious problems in my marriage." To focus on the child without considering the husband-wife relationship is sometimes counter-productive because a frequent cause of a child's problem stems from his mother and father's relationship.

All the elements that have been suggested for a healthy one-to-one parent-child relationship, i.e., understanding, the stages of learning, attitudes and motivation, time, instruction, sharing, disclosure, and empathy, are important for the most sacred of all one-to-one relationships. If the husband-wife relationship is intact, the prognosis for happy, fulfilled parents and children is good.

An Alternative to Therapy

Many men and women find comfort and release in a one-to-one relationship with a therapist because the relationship gives them a time and place in which they can ventilate their feelings and share their thoughts without being judged. They know they can open themselves in this way because their disclosures will be treated in confidence by someone who cares and who does not reprimand them. The whole environment exists to solve problems, not create them.

In all probability, there will always be a need for such client-therapist relationships. But the need for therapists would be radically decreased if the same environment created by them for the benefit of their clients were to be translated to the home by informed and caring parents. If the 41 per cent of all parents who reported parenting to be a negative experience were to create such an atmosphere of love and caring in their homes, they might turn what has been until now a frustrating experience into the most exciting of all human relationships.

Finally, there is "something special and sacred" about the relationship between two people that is lost when three, four, or more are involved. There is time to learn, to look, to listen, to feel, to share, to enjoy, to plan, and to resolve. It's a fundamental relationship that can cement, heal, and build for the future. It's a set of skills that must be learned, and when these skills are learned the payoffs are forever: for early and middle childhood, for the bumpy adolescence, and for a strong mature friendship beyond the caretaking years.

FIVE

Good Kids, Bad Kids, and Parent Expectations

Children rarely question our expectations; instead they question their personal adequacy.

— DOROTHY CORKVILLE BRIGGS

The difference between a lady and a flower girl is not how she behaves but how she is treated. I shall always be a flower girl to Professor Higgins because he always treats me as a flower girl and always will; but I know I can be a lady to you because you always treat me as a lady and always will.

— LIZA DOLITTLE, IN G.B. SHAW'S *PYGMALION*

The Self-fulfilling Prophecy

Expectations are powerful determinants of our behaviour and the behaviour of our children. Expectations can build or destroy. A team of Harvard scientists has studied the role and the effects of expectations and concluded that most individuals do what is expected of them either as a function of their own or others' expectations. Predictions and expectations determine an individual's attitude and experiences. Experiments have demonstrated that the sweet can taste sweeter, the bitter more bitter, and the sweet can become sour, depending on one's expectations.

In my experience with parent-teacher conflicts, often a parent's anticipation that a teacher will be difficult and unco-operative leads the parents to turn hostile or defensive. This, in turn, leads to a self-fulfilling prophecy: a conflict between parent and teacher, which in the end hurts the child.

Professor Robert Rosenthal of Harvard, in his studies of teachers' expectations of pupils' intellectual competence, found that the teachers' initial expectations could actually form and shape the students' competence. When teachers were told that a specific group of children had unusually high potential, and in fact the names of the children in this group were just randomly picked out of a hat, the pupils in this special group showed substantial increases in I.Q. The teachers' expectations of the specific group (who were no different from the rest of the class) actually led to significant gains in their intellectual performance. Other investigations have shown that teachers with high expectations give such pupils more time, attention, and encouragement, and in turn receive more positive feedback. Since teachers have a limited amount of time, pupils for whom the teacher had low expectations were not given comparable time, attention, and reinforcement, and thus turned in poorer performances.

It has been found that many teachers base their expectations on previous records of ability or performance. If a pupil had one difficult year, he would thus pay for it for the rest of his educational career. Past records can generate many problems, leading to poor teaching, slow motivation, a deprived environment, or illnesses. Previous records may give some direction, but they should not form the basis for inflexible conclusions or unwarranted expectations. Teachers' expectations are also based at times on racial prejudices. Does the child come from a white, middle-class family? Is his skin dark? Is his family on welfare? These and like expectations determine their teaching behaviour. Prejudice and stereotypes lead to expectations, and the expectations in turn determine behaviour.

It has been well-documented in sports that when an athlete fears or expects failure, he fails. His expectation of failure creates over-anxiety, which in turn affects his concentration, his co-ordination, and the intensity of his effort. Similar findings on the costs of expectations are found in industry, in social situations, and even in such mundane activities as driving a car. Thousands of studies in psychosomatic medicine give us added evidence that negative expectations can make you sick or sicker, while positive expectations can help to heal.

"Good Kids and Bad Kids"

Parents who expect "bad" or negative behaviour from their children inevitably find it. Some children can never erase a bad behaviour from their record – they have been sentenced. The expectations of bad behaviour create a self-fulfilling prophecy and the parents' reactions can cause negative behaviour. *It's important to expect and "catch" good behaviour.*

Parents who have high expectations that are in line with a child's capacity and goals usually see their expectations fulfilled. Just as with the teachers in the Harvard study, the expectations of such parents actually make good things happen. These parents attain more because they put more stress on positive relationships and give more positive reinforcement, time, and direction to their children. The converse is also true: a parent's low expectations can dull a child's ambition and limit a child's progress.

If a parents' expectations are self-serving, self-indulging, and insensitive to a child's abilities and interests, they can do serious damage. The cases of Paul N. and Peter J., from our files, illustrate the costs of parental expectations.

ONLY SISSIES CRY: THE CASE OF PAUL N.

Paul's parents were concerned because he was effeminate. He didn't play with boys and had only one friend – a girl. They were troubled because Paul didn't participate in sports but preferred to read or to write poetry and plays. Up to the age of seven, he would play with dolls and dress up in his sister's clothes. Paul, who was ten, was short for his age and about ten pounds overweight.

His father was extremely disturbed about Paul's appearance, his feminine behaviour, and his tendency to cry. "When I was a youngster my dad would whack the hell out of me if I cried," said the father. "He would say, 'The Lord never meant boys to cry – only sissies cry.'" Mr. N. professed to be a very religious person, and in our conversations, whenever he wanted to emphasize a point, he would invoke the name of God. Mr. N. was a six-foot-two-inch, all-around athlete – an excellent skier, hunter, sailor, and golfer. The house motto was "mens sana in corpore sano." For him, a sound mind only existed in a sound body, and sports was the pathway to both. "Paul's mind and body are not developing properly because he doesn't take part in sports."

Mr. N. had taken Paul duck-hunting one fall. As they sat in the blind with the rain pouring down, Paul began to cry "I want to go home!" Mr. N. hit him, and Paul began to sob hysterically, and to shiver, and couldn't catch his breath. Mr. N. became terribly upset. He just couldn't understand this child. The incident so troubled Mr. N. that he decided to consult the family physician regarding his concerns about Paul's effeminate behaviour and Paul's reaction to a "mere slap." The physician in turn referred him to us for psychological consultation.

Paul went through a battery of tests and interviews. He was found to be extremely bright, congenial, articulate, and creative, but his anxiety level was very high. He had difficulty sleeping for fear of bed-wetting and felt guilty and confused about his love-hate feelings toward his father. He was also somewhat confused by his mother, who alternated between over-protectiveness on the one hand and threats of withdrawal of her love and of physical punishment on the other. Though Paul had somehow survived this corrosive home environment, we were concerned with the fact that much of his writing focused on suicide. Fantasy so often often precedes reality.

Paul's major support was a female music teacher at school. He would share with her his innermost thoughts, his poetry, his music, his sadness, and his guilt. She gave him the affection and encouragement he needed so badly. Late at night he would often fantasize that the teacher was his mother, or his girl friend.

In all our interviews, Paul never criticized his parents, never considered that they were wrong. He felt *he* was wrong, and that he was a terrible disappointment to them. In one of our weekly sessions, Paul and I played a game called "Magic Man" where I could grant him any wish, but only one wish. He wished for a brother.

H.M.: What would your brother be like?

PAUL: He would be a super skier, hockey player, football player, and win lots of ribbons and medals.

H.M.: I suppose that having such a brother would take the pressure off you?

PAUL: Not really, I would like a brother, because I'm not what my Dad wants.

Because all our discussions were confidential, I asked Paul for his permission to tell his father about our "Magic Man" game. He said it would be all right with him.

At our next interview with Mr. N., Paul's father again made a remark to the effect that when God created man he did not intend man to cry. I suggested that God, in his wisdom, would not have given the man the equipment to cry if he did not want him to cry, and that perhaps God felt that crying could serve as a stress release, a safety valve, for men as it does for women. He had never thought about it like that and conceded that perhaps it might be so. He would have to think about it. I then told him about the "Magic Man" episode and, for the first time, Mr. N. choked up and did not look at me directly. I talked with him further.

H.M.: Your son loves you, is different from you, and is in a great deal of pain because of it. Should he be? He is a tremendously creative youngster. Have you ever read any of his poetry or his plays? Many of our great poets and playwrights were male. They were not less male because of these interests. We don't think that Paul has a male identity problem. He sees himself as a boy, but his interpretation of boyness may be different from yours. Your attitude and your pressure are really confusing him.

MR. N.: Are you suggesting that I'm responsible for his problems? For his feminine behaviour?

H.M.: You will have to decide what your nonacceptance has done to him and whether it is responsible for his feelings of anxiety, guilt, and failure as a son. Is it possible that he avoids sports because of your high expectations and super abilities in sport? He doesn't feel he could win ribbons and medals. Don't you really wish he could? By never having shared his creativity, never having listened to his poetry and plays, have you perhaps not rejected him? What are the consequences of your attempting to subdue his individuality so that he may fulfil your expectations? How must he feel in an environment of rejection and derision, and what are his alternatives? Your son is a very special youngster to have survived as well as he has.

In the next few months Mr. and Mrs. N. wrestled with their expectations and their values, and very slowly began to explore Paul's world. And very slowly they also began to enjoy his special gifts and accept his uniqueness.

Paul is now twelve; the anxiety, guilt, and bed-wetting are past history. Paul has developed an interest in tennis. The pressure is off, now that he is no longer threatened. And in this new climate of acceptance, he can explore his father's world as his father explores his.

This case had a good ending. Many don't.

DRUGS AND CARPENTRY: THE CASE OF PETER J.

Peter's father was a physician, his mother a school teacher. They came into the office and – before I could ask why they had come – Mrs. J. opened up in a very firm, authoritative manner:

This is what I would like you to do. Peter is sixteen, has dropped out of twelfth grade, is experimenting with drugs, and sometimes stays away from home for a week at a time. He has agreed to come to see you. I would like you to, first, convince him to go back to school and, second, convince him of the importance of training for a profession. We don't care whether he goes into medicine, law, or engineering – that's his choice; but he must go to university. He is very bright and should not waste his abilities. You must also point out to him the dangers of drug abuse; he is just not listening to us. If he carries on this way he is going to destroy himself and us. This situation is beyond us and we can't handle it. It's affecting our work, our marriage, and our total life.

For fifteen years Peter was a terrific youngster, excellent at school, had lots of friends, enjoyed sports, and was great around the house. And then one day last June he told us he wanted to register in a vocational school to specialize in woodworking and become a master carpenter.

We said we couldn't go along with that decision, and that he had the ability to go to university. We told him we were prepared to finance his education to become a doctor or whatever profession he decided on. I pointed out that, as a teacher, I was aware of the intellectual and academic level of kids that end up in a vocational school; that it was a dumping ground for the slow learners, the behavioural problems, and the delinquents. A trade was a dead end for those short on brains or who couldn't afford a university career.

After many discussions which usually ended up in heated shouting matches, Peter said, "If I can't go to vocational school and become a carpenter and do what I want to do, I'm going to quit school and get a job."

We thought that doing this might be good for him and teach him a lesson on how difficult it is to make money. We thought also that Peter would discover, by working, that the workingman's environment would be a deadening one for him.

He got a job as a waiter in a restaurant where he met some characters who introduced him to the dope scene. His father, being a physician, has over the years talked with Peter about the dangers of drugs. He has told us that he is not into any hard stuff, and that 60 per cent of the population smokes pot. We're really concerned about his psychological dependency on drugs. Can you help us?

Though Mrs. J. had begun with an authoritative set of instructions, she ended with a plaintive plea for help. I finally got a chance to respond to her torrent of preconceived notions.

H.M.: It seems that the situation developed because you refused to support his decision to become a carpenter. What are your objections to carpentry as an occupation?

MRS. J.: I don't object to carpentry. It so happens that Dr. J.'s hobby is woodworking, and Peter and he have made some great furniture for the house. That's where he got the bug. But that's where it should stay – just a hobby. Do you have children?

H.M.: Yes, I have three daughters.

MRS. J.: Well, what if one of them, instead of going to university to get an education, decided to go to a hairdressing college. How would you feel? Not to be a snob, but if some of your friends should ask, "What is your daughter doing now?" would you feel comfortable with, "She's a hairdresser?"

H.M.: Let's examine some of your assumptions: first, that only people who go to university are educated and, second, that if you go to university you come out educated. I teach at a university and have found that many students pass in and out without absorbing an education. Being a carpenter doesn't preclude being educated. Peter's interest in woodworking and his creativity, combined with the learning of basic and advanced skills, could possibly lead, for example, to his making an important contribution in the world of furniture design.

You can become educated with a library card. Education is the result of an attitude, not a place. You're right – I would prefer my daughter to be a doctor or lawyer rather than a hairdresser, and I have the right to state this and encourage her, but I do not have the right to demand that she fulfil *my* expectations, *my* values, and *my* needs. I could destroy her, or ruin our relationship, by trying to legislate. As a parent I can suggest, I can advise, but if I have been a competent parent, I would have taught her how to evaluate her own abilities and needs and how to make her own decisions. She is not just an extension of me. She is a unique, separate personality with her own private set of values and motives, and it's her privilege to decide what she wants to do with her life.

Over the next few months, in family sessions that included Peter, his father and mother began to assess the costs of their expectations. They had lost their precious relationship with Peter, which had been warm, loving, open, and filled with so many shared adventures and discoveries. They had always trusted Peter, but somewhere along the line – in the heat of their expectations – they had forgotten to trust him.

The road to listening and to acceptance was painful, but they recognized their priorities and listened. Much of what they heard from Peter finally convinced them that their son could shoulder his own problems, make his own decisions, and become an independent person. They also clearly heard his plea for their continued trust and support. Their relationship entered a new stage.

After a number of sessions, Dr. and Mrs. J. and their son worked out an understanding, "a contract," under which Peter, after family consultation, would make the final decision. Peter quit his job in the restaurant and for extra money worked Saturdays in his father's laboratory. In the fall he enrolled in a carpentry course at the vocational school.

Three years have passed. Peter is now twenty-one. He completed his training in woodworking, won a furniture-design award, worked for one year as an apprentice carpenter, and has now decided he would like to study medical engineering. He is taking make-up courses in math and science and intends to enrol in a university program.

Not all cases end on an upbeat note, as Paul's and Peter's did. Many children's lives are irreversibly damaged by their parents' unreal expectations.

The Anatomy of Expectations

The cases of Peter and Paul illustrate how potentially powerful and destructive parental expectations can be, how they can confuse, damage, and destroy relationships. Often, a parent's expectations for a child say more about the parent's needs, values, and personality than about the child's.

Research studies have found that parents are quite accurate in *assessing* and *estimating* their child's social, intellectual, verbal, and physical abilities. However, parents often seem to lose the capacity for accurate assessment when they try to set goals for their children. When their expectations are really nothing more than an expression of their own needs, then conflicts and disappointments can follow for both parent and child. These conflicts and disappointments in turn can breed an atmosphere of negativism that slows or stops the child's growth and development.

We see many children in our clinics who, because of their failure to meet their parents' expectations, manifest symptoms of hyperactivity, gastro-intestinal disorders, neuroses, phobias, bed-wetting, rejection of the school system, and delinquency. Misplaced or unreasonable expectations are rarely intentional. They are usually the product of intense feelings and convictions, and of lack of awareness of the probable consequences. On the other hand, realistic expectations can build, motivate, and encourage a child. If expectations are in harmony with a child's abilities and needs, then they will excite and reinforce the child's own motives and efforts. If expectations are explained clearly, they can serve to give the child guidelines and direction. Reasonable expectations say "I care" and "I have confidence in you."

How do we keep our expectations realistic and thus avoid damage? I think it begins with an understanding of the *anatomy* of our expectations. What are the elements of an expectation? What are the factors that affect or determine our expectations? How do we modify them and utilize them for the ultimate good of our children?

THE ELEMENTS OF AN EXPECTATION

"I expect Rebecca to be a great concert pianist."
"I expect Lloyd to be a minister."
"I expect Charlie to share his toys with other kids."

"I expect Elizabeth to marry a Catholic and have at least four children."

All of the above expectations include three common elements: a set of *beliefs*, a set of *feelings*, and a set of *actions*. For example, "I expect Rebecca to be a great concert pianist" may mean that: (1) you believe she is very talented and has an aptitude for music, or that piano is a great career; (2) you would be excited by her success, and it would give you great joy and satisfaction to hear her perform in London, Paris, and Rome, thus fulfilling an ardent, long-standing dream; and (3) that you would engage the best piano teachers, send her to Europe for training, and see to it that she practises, practises, and practises.

The most powerful element that determines *actions* is not one's belief, but one's *feelings*. Even though you may finally discover that Rebecca is tone deaf and has poor hand-eye co-ordination, your intense motivation and your ardent feelings haven't changed. You may ignore your beliefs and take her from teacher to teacher, hoping someone will work a miracle. This is called "magical expectation," and it can lead to deep frustrations.

It's important to understand and to be sensitive to these three elements of expectation because, even though you may be intellectually rational about an expectation, your feelings may cloud your ability to judge realistically.

FACTORS THAT AFFECT YOUR EXPECTATIONS

Your religion, parents' values and expectations, education, job, financial status, social status, friends, abilities, personality (self-esteem), and the media all can affect your values, motives, feelings, and interests. These in turn affect your expectations of your children. If your child shows talent for or interest in languages, music, art, or athletics, your expectations are influenced.

Your child's expectations and goals will affect your expectations of him. If he decides to go to university to become an engineer, your expectations may be in agreement. If, however, he decides that he wants to become a ballet dancer, your expectations for him may not be in agreement. In addition, comparisons with other children in terms of their rate of development and their accomplishments may set up expectations that may or may not be appropriate for your child. If your next-door neighbour's child walks at the age of fifteen months and has a vocabulary of 400 words at the age of two, these attainments may tempt you to expect comparable performances of your child. If yours doesn't live up to this expectation, your impatience may put pressure on the

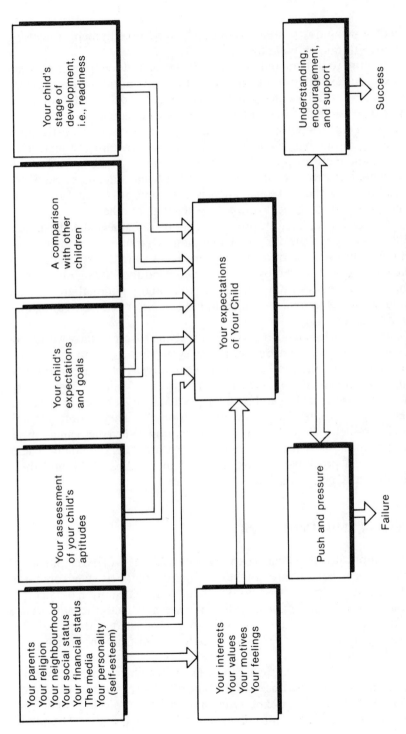

Figure 7. Factors Affecting Parental Expectations

79

child, slowing down rather than accelerating development or causing emotional trauma along the way.

Failure to understand your child's stages of development also can affect your expectations. Children go through various stages of development physically, emotionally, intellectually, socially, and morally. And there are individual differences between children in their rates of development. Though all children pass through all the stages in the same order, each one has his own timetable for progression through these stages, and there are limits to the extent to which parents can affect this individual growth schedule. Attainment of one stage is essential for "readiness" for the next stage. There is no skipping of stages. Sometimes one facet of development proceeds faster than another.

For example, Kevin is only fifteen years old and is already six feet tall with the physique of a grown man, but his emotions and intellectual equipment are those of a fifteen-year-old. A parent's expectations of Kevin may be distorted by his physical appearance. Being unaware of the differing rates of physical, intellectual, and emotional growth can induce parents to make mistakes in judgement or action, creating and sometimes ensuring failure.

In the little leagues of baseball, hockey, and soccer we have witnessed the sad results of excessive expectations by overly anxious and ambitious fathers. Some of these fathers – without being aware of it – are vicariously enjoying athletic competition through their sons. Many of these youngsters who are forced to endure 6 a.m. practice sessions are not mature neurologically, physically, and/or emotionally. They simply are not ready for such intense training and competition. When they cannot meet Dad's expectations, there is disappointment, pressure, and failure. These failures can prove contagious, affecting their school work and their family and social relationships.

Stages of Moral Development

The importance of matching expectations with stages of development or readiness can be seen through the examination of the six stages of moral development. None of us is born with an immediate notion of fairness, ethics, justice, sharing, or morality. We are born with the *capacity* to learn these concepts and the behaviour associated with them. The learning comes primarily from our parents and from the society into which we are born.

At what age or stage, then, can we expect a child to share for the sake of sharing and to help others for the sake of helping – rather than simply for barter? When can we expect a child to consider the feelings of others? When does a child begin to understand justice and fairness? (Andrew will not share his toys! Cynthia lets her brother use her skates – for ten cents! Bill steals money from the family cookie jar. When will he learn to be honest?)

According to world-renowned child psychologist Jean Piaget, morality develops when a child understands and accepts social rules, and when he is concerned about equality, justice, and reciprocity in human relationships. This moral maturity is possible only when a child's intellectual equipment has matured, and not until then. Professor Kohlberg suggests six stages through which we must pass before we develop Piaget's notion of morality.

Stage 1. In this stage, children learn to obey their parents to avoid punishment. Rules are immutable, and are made by the parents who hold the power. Morality at this stage is defined in terms of the physical consequences of disobedience. (Note: many adults have become fixated at this first stage: their only reason to obey rules is to avoid punishment. They never advance beyond this rudimentary level, however old they get.)

Stage 2. Children now conform to rules to gain rewards. Sharing is practised for selfish and self-rewarding reasons, not out of generosity. It's bartering time – "You can use my bat, if you give me your popsicle."

Stage 3. Conforming at this stage is for social approval rather than in exchange for things or for the avoidance of physical punishment. Social disapproval is the chief punishment at this stage.

Stage 4. There is a recognition of rules beyond the rules at home. There is recognition and conformity to society's rules, and the conformity is sometimes rigid. Most people stop growing at this stage.

Stage 5. This is a more mature stage of morality, marked by recognition of individual rights and democratic law and by agreement to maintain the social order and the rights of individuals. There is also a flexibility in moral beliefs and social contracts which can be modified by rationally discussing alternatives. Obedience to rules is not always held to be necessary, and violation is not held always to be wrong.

Stage 6. This is the optimal stage of moral development. Morality is based on respect for self and others. There is a development of internalized rules and belief in equal justice for all.

HOW DOES THIS MORALITY COME ABOUT?

To a certain extent the stages of moral development may be age-related, but they are primarily determined by the stages of mental development. We can't expect a five-year-old to attain the fourth or fifth stage because he just does not have the intellectual abilities necessary to understand such notions as individual rights and social order. We must wait until his mental equipment matures before we can reasonably expect more mature behaviour.

An understanding of social justice comes with intellectual development, as well as with the development of independence and the growth of self-esteem, and through interaction with peers. Most of all it comes from parental example. When parents move from their traditional position of unilateral authority and attempt to establish equal relationships with their children, they accelerate the final two stages and the acquisition of reciprocal morality and justice.

As Professor Kohlberg points out, many parents are themselves fixated at earlier stages of moral development, and their fixation puts a ceiling on their children's moral and ethical growth. High expectations for stages five and six can only come about if parents conform to the same rules as they impose on their children and set examples by establishing a home climate of self-respect, respect for others, and justice. Some parents cannot cope with changes in command, with the gradual lessening of the authority structure and an acceptance of the child's growth toward independence; thus they force an adolescent to "fight or flee."

In sum, if you expect moral behaviour of your child, you must first understand the stage of readiness of your child to behave in the expected manner and, also, you must teach by example the behaviour you expect. Understanding the stages of development – physical, intellectual, emotional, social, and moral – gives a parent some direction as to what are reasonable expectations.

How to Change or Modify Your Expectations

Learning to change our expectations is very difficult for a number of reasons.

1. They are so entrenched in the values of our society.

2. Our conscious and subconscious expectations are promoted and exploited by the media.

3. We learn them when we are young and unquestioning.

4. They serve very strong and sometimes selfish motives. After years of learning and overlearning expectations become almost like reflexes. For example, many newlyweds plan to have children because it's a societal expectation they have adopted as their own. In this instance, their motives are not necessarily related to a genuine love of children.

5. If we finally do realize that some of our expectations are unfair, the "belief component" of our expectation may change or be modified.

But the feeling or "emotional component" is often much slower to change. Our behaviour continues to be affected by our feelings more than by our beliefs. By being in touch with and aware of our deep feelings we can begin to recognize them as "controlling feelings."

CONFLICTING EXPECTATIONS

Many of our expectations come in bunches or constellations and are determined by religion or by some specific segment of society. If you are born Catholic, your attitudes and expectations about whom you marry and where, who conducts the service, and about abortion and divorce are all part of a constellation of Catholic expectations. If you are born very rich, you will have certain expectations regarding education, dress, achievement, whom you marry, and where you should live.

Some expectations conflict within the person or within the culture and create problems. According to research studies, most people in our culture still hold stereotyped expectations for boys. "I expect my boy to be active, strong, good at sports, independent, unemotional, and aggressive." The problem with this expectation is that it often conflicts with the expectations of those who dominate the school culture. "A student should sit quietly in his seat, be neat, pay attention, and be interested in reading, writing, and arithmetic."

Virginia Sexton, in her research on thousands of high school students, found that boys who scored high on a test of masculinity scored low on educational achievement tests. A number of problems have resulted from the differences between the expectations of *boy culture* and *school culture*. Almost 80 per cent of all children with learning and delinquency problems are boys. Some researchers feel this imbalance is due in part to these incompatible expectations.

CHECK YOUR EXPECTATIONS

Parental expectations can have a salutary effect, and they can encourage and motivate. They must, however, be realistic. They must be communicated to the child and be consonant with his own expectations. The following Parent Expectation Check List may help to identify and rate your own expectations.

Parent Expectation Check List
1. Identify and list your expectations clearly.
2. Rate the importance to you of each expectation on a scale of 1 to 10. 10 is an expectation that is very important, and 1 is unimportant.
3. List your five most important expectations in the order of importance.

4. What are you doing to help your child achieve?
5. Have you declared these expectations clearly to your child?
6. What are your spouse's expectations?
7. Does he/she declare them clearly and openly?
8. What does he/she do about them?
9. Are there any differences between your spouse's expectations and yours?
10. If there are differences, what is the effect of these differences and how do you resolve them?
11. Can you identify your child's expectations? List them.
12. Rate your perception of their importance to your child.
13. Are they similar to your expectations?
14. What is your estimate of your child's present level of functioning and potential in each of the following categories?

	Below Average		Average		Above Average	
	Present Level	Potential	Present Level	Potential	Present Level	Potential
a) intellectual						
b) academic						
c) social						
d) moral, ethical						
e) language						
f) physical skills						
g) artistic skills						
h) personality						
i)						
j)						

15. Are your expectations of your child in line with the above assessment of your child's level of functioning?

Many parents have found this check list very helpful for a number of reasons. (1) Many of our expectations are just below the surface of awareness (or denial). By trying to identify and rate them, we begin to better understand our own behaviour and its consequences for our children. (2) Openly declaring your expectations produces a family environment of honesty and trust. (3) Differences in expectations between parent and child, and between parents as they affect the child, explain a great deal about parental and child behaviour. Seeing these differences is essential prior to discussing them. Discussion provides the possibility of resolution. (4) By listing our expectations, we often begin to see contradictions within our own sets of expectations and between our estimate of a child's capacity or ability and our expectations. (5) Any organization or team operates better when it has a common goal and when energies are not diluted by the push-pull and agony of conflicting views. Similarly, congruity, or agreement on expectations between parent and parent and between parent and child, increases the probability of success. (6) As your children grow and mature your expectations must be secondary to their expectations. Successful achievement and satisfaction with this achievement will depend on their assumption of their own problems and their decision as to the direction of their lives.

Finally, one of the obligations that comes with the privilege of declaring our expectations for our children is the obligation to provide parental direction, example, and encouragement. An expectation usually denotes moving from one level of behaviour to another, from one level of achievement to a higher level. In travelling this route from lower to higher expectations, it helps to have a road map. Since parents have travelled some of these routes themselves, they can help the younger traveller by pointing out what the road looks like, the potholes and detours, the points of interest and the necessary preparations.

SIX

Don't Step on My Self-concept

You are my mirror. I see myself as you see me.
Accept me as I am and I will accept myself.

Verbal Whips, Fantasy, and Stomach Aches: The Case of Roger P.

Roger, a nine-year-old, was having difficulty in school. He had repeated grade two and was about two years behind in reading. The school psychologist reported that he had an average I.Q. but was not motivated. He was a loner, watched about twenty-six hours of TV a week, complained of headaches, stomach pains, and difficulty with his breathing, and fantasized and daydreamed a great deal. His family doctor diagnosed his symptoms as psychosomatic. His parents had tried tutors, changing his teacher, three pediatricians, megavitamins, behaviour management for a month, and spanking without any success.

Within the first two minutes of our first interview, Mother told Roger to sit up, stop slouching, leave his nose alone, and pay attention. Whenever Roger answered one of my questions either Mother or Father would correct him, telling him he was wrong or that it was a lie. Dad kept referring to his laziness, lack of motivation, and hiding behind his mother or the television set whenever things had to be done. When I asked them what they liked about Roger, the father answered, "Right now – nothing! He is really going to have to change his ways before we can say anything good!"

I kept wondering how all these comments were affecting Roger and whether he had developed a turn-off mechanism by going into his fantasy life and daydreams. Their "put-downs" showed no sensitivity, no regard for Roger's self-esteem. They seemed to reach for put-downs to justify their assessment of Roger's "badness." Whatever the original cause might have been for Roger's school failure, e.g., lack of neurological or language readiness, poor teaching, or a school phobia, the parents were helping by their constant put-downs to nail the lid on his growth and progress. They were destroying the most central element of Roger's personality, his self-concept – the element that mobilizes, energizes, motivates, and maintains stability in the face of difficulties. What a dilemma! Failure and embarrassment at school, no friends, verbal abuse and sometimes physical abuse at home. After a while, "you're bad, you're lazy, you don't pay attention, you're a failure, you lie," plus his failures academically, socially, and familially, convince Roger "I am a failure! I am bad!" To escape from all this pain and frustration, Roger turns to headaches and stomach pains because for a moment it diverts and he receives a little consolation from his mother. He escapes into his fantasies and daydreams where he can be anything and succeed. It's a better place than his painful reality. The problem with such escapism is that it becomes comfortable, and a neurotic habit.

Often I feel that it's the parents who should have been referred. If they did not create the original problem of school failure, they were maintaining and magnifying it. Roger's self-concept had bottomed and was continually being confirmed by his parents. In our first two-hour session they scored at least fifty put-downs, such as:

- You're rude!
- You're not listening!
- What's the matter with you?
- He's just lazy.
- He's old enough to know better.
- How many times have I told you ...?
- You are going to end up nowhere!
- That's a stupid comment!
- That's no reason to cry.
- etc.

When the session was over, the father said, "And now I hope you appreciate what we have to put up with." Poor, bad Roger, the prosecuting attorneys had presented a very damaging case.

Was Roger's original school problem unusual? Were his parent's reactions to his failure and his subsequent behaviour unusual? Was this case just a case to dramatically make a point? Most children and most parents are not really like that! Are they? The incidence of psychological problems is so great in today's society that few families escape without being affected. Millions of children and adults have learning and emotional problems. *The unusual has become the usual.* Do Roger's parents understand how vulnerable a child's self-concept is, that a self-concept determines what we think, how we feel, and what we do about ourselves? Parents, after all, are the most important agents in the early development of a child's self-concept, and a child's self-concept becomes fixed and determines the adult's self-concept and his success and failures.

What Is a Self-concept?

Is our self-concept determined by our genes? Is it learned? What is a healthy self-concept? How does it develop? Who and what affects the growth of a healthy self-concept? How does it affect our everyday functioning and lifestyle? Can it be modified or changed? How?

Our self-concept is what we think we are, and what we think other people think we are. It is, as Byrne suggests, "the total collection of attitudes, judgements, and values which an individual holds with respect to his behaviour, his abilities, his body, his worth as a person – in short, how he perceives and evaluates himself." It is our internal picture of ourself. A positive self-concept is essential for our mental health, social competence, personal happiness, adjustment, and effective functioning.

A self-concept is learned from infancy to adulthood; it is not determined by our genes. We begin with a clean slate and what is written on this self-concept slate comes from the feedback we get from our parents, families, friends, teachers, the society in which we live, and from our evaluation of our experiences. "We value ourselves as we are valued by others." Messages about ourselves come to us through many channels verbally in terms of statements of acceptance and praise or statements of derision and criticism, visually through facial expressions that may reflect approval and warmth or disdain and disgust, and physically through a hug, a pat on the back, or through a slap or pinch. Symbolic messages also affect our self-concept. They come to us through grades, marks, promotions, titles, and labels. We have a sensitive radar system always on the alert to pick up these messages that help us fill in this complex jigsaw puzzle – our self-concept. Though it is a lifetime quest, the basis for much of the self-concept develops by the age of five and becomes quite stable by the age of twelve to eighteen.

The self-concept is all-powerful, for it influences all our behaviour in terms of success and failure and is the most critical indicator of our stability and mental health. It is not a simple personality trait but a very complex and intricate system. Before we begin to tinker with it we should understand its anatomy, its parts, its characteristics, how it grows, what it affects, and how to change it.

A self-concept is composed of several sub-self-concepts, which combine to make up the whole self-concept. At one time we thought there was only one self-concept and that it determined whether you really felt good or poorly about yourself, in *all* situations. Researchers have discovered that we own a number of different self-concepts and that, though interrelated, they can operate separately. Thus, we have a physical self-concept, a personal self-concept, a social self-concept, a family self-concept, an ethical-moral self-concept, and an achievement (school or work) self-concept.

- A *physical self-concept* is made up of our evaluation of our physical skills, fitness, sexuality, state of health, and physical appearance.
- A *social self-concept* is our evaluation of how we function in relationship with other people and in various social situations.
- A *family self-concept* is our evaluation of how we get along with family members and how we fit into the family, i.e., our status in the family and our sense of adequacy as a family member.
- A *moral-ethical self-concept* is our evaluation of our moral, religious, and ethical values and behaviour and can indicate our contribution to society.
- A *personal self-concept* is our own evaluation of our personality, personal worth, and self-confidence.
- A *school or work self-concept* is our evaluation of our functioning and achievements in academic or vocational settings.

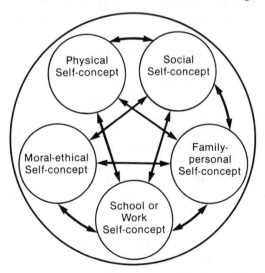

Figure 8. The Whole Self-concept and Sub-self-concepts

The value of this conceptualization of self-concepts is that we can, by an analysis of these various subselves, get a better understanding of the total self. For example, it is possible to have a high physical self-concept and a low social self-concept or a high work self-concept and a low physical self-concept. If parents are sensitive, listen, and observe carefully, they can pick up messages that will give them information about these different self-concepts as well as some direction to help with a child's low self-concepts.

For example, consider ten-year-old Tony, who feels very good about his school self: his marks are excellent and his teacher likes him. But he feels very uncomfortable about his physical self and his social self. He is very poor at baseball: no one ever chooses him, he is always left on the bench, and he begins to avoid going out to play with the other kids who seem to avoid him. His parents can't understand it because he is so pleasant at home and good at school.

There is no automatic spread effect or transference from one self-concept to another. Tony may know how to solve a math problem, but he can't catch, throw, run, or hit a ball. Are these skills really necessary to be accepted? If the social activity among his peers is baseball, it is necessary and he needs some help with the development of his ball playing skills. If he doesn't get some help, he will avoid the embarrassment of failure and may become a loner. What are his alternatives?

Most children pick up these skills gradually and easily, but some have a slower motor and perceptual-motor rate of development. They have problems with hand-eye co-ordination, balance, rhythm, and reaction time. Because of early failures they avoid and never build up these deficits and the necessary strength and stamina needed for physical involvement. In the early years, perhaps more so for boys than girls, physical involvement such as sports is *the* social activity for that age group.

Tony's options involve an exchange arrangement with someone who is good at sports but needs help with his math. Peer tutors are sometimes the most effective. Another option includes an analysis of what Tony is capable of, a breakdown of the baseball skills requirements into small chunks, and an opportunity to learn these chunks or bits in a one-to-one situation with his father or another family member or a friend. When he does have this repertoire of skills, he will have a better concept of his physical self and the confidence to begin to play with the other boys.

An interesting finding from our work with children who have socialization problems is that some of these children, because of either a lack of opportunity or slow physical maturation, get lost in large physical education classes and receive less attention and less reinforcement than the children who are succeeding, and consequently they fall further and further behind. Their frustration and embarrassment result in avoidance. In a non-threatening one-to-one situation, when assisted with the basic and necessary physical and sport skills, they were able to enter into the physical-social activities. Of course, other factors also influence social competencies, but as we have seen, physical self-concept in children is closely related to their social self-concept.

THE THREE BASIC PARTS OF A SELF-CONCEPT

A self-concept is an attitude about yourself, and to be able to understand and try to improve, you must understand what it is made up of, i.e., its three parts: facts or beliefs, feelings, and behaviour. *Facts or beliefs* about ourselves describe who we are. We may believe that we are tall, or fat, or considerate, or religious, or bright, or physically well co-ordinated. From others and our experiences we develop this set of beliefs. *Feelings* and emotions about ourselves indicate: I am anxious, or fearful, or guilty, or happy. "I feel good about myself," or "I hate myself." *Behaviours* describe what an individual does or how he acts and whether he approaches or avoids situations. "I'm going to watch TV because I don't have any friends to play with."

Attitudes are difficult to change. That is primarily so because it has been assumed that an attitude is *only* made up of a set of beliefs, facts, and information, and that to change or modify an attitude and behaviour all we have to do is to supply new information and facts. From our research on attitudes regarding obesity, overweight, physical fitness, and prejudices, however, we have found that additional facts and information do not necessarily lead to a change. We have missed one of the keys to attitude change: the *feeling* component. You can change a negative belief to a positive belief, but unless you change the *negative feelings* to *positive feelings* there will be little change in behaviour.

Consider, for example, the possibilities in your attitude to Mr. X.

(1) If your beliefs and your feelings about Mr. X are negative your behaviour toward Mr. X will be negative, that is, you will avoid him. (2) If your beliefs and feelings are positive about Mr. X your behaviour will be positive; you will be nice and approach Mr. X. (3) If your beliefs are positive, but your feelings about Mr. X are negative, you will probably be uncomfortable and avoid him. (4) If your beliefs about Mr. X are negative, but your feelings about him are positive, that is, you feel good and comfortable with him, your behaviour will be positive and you will want to be with him in spite of your negative beliefs. In short, then, feelings are powerful – check them out!

EXAMPLES OF THE THREE PARTS OF A SELF-CONCEPT

Example 1 – My Physical Self-concept

My Belief – I am fat, nothing fits, and it's a glandular problem.

My Feeling – I *hate* myself. I am *embarrassed* by my appearance.

My Behaviour – I avoid social gatherings, sports, my friends, my family, and I gorge myself.

Example 2 – My Social Self-concept

My Belief – I don't know what to say to people. I am not interesting. People ignore me at parties.

My Feeling – I feel tense and very fearful in social situations. I become very self-conscious and nervous.

My Behaviour – I avoid meeting people or going to any social gatherings.

Example 3 – My School Self-concept

My Belief – I am an excellent student, good at math, science, and languages.

My Feeling – I enjoy school. I enjoy reading. I am happy and proud of my A's.

My Behaviour – I am taking extra courses. I am tutoring and exploring various university programs.

Example 4 – My Moral-Ethical Self-concept

My Belief – I am a liar and I cheat.

My Feeling – I really feel guilty and fearful that someone will find out.

My Behaviour – I keep on lying to cover up my previous lies.

Example 5 – My Personal Self-concept

My Belief – I have a great sense of humour.

My Feeling – I enjoy people's reaction to my stories and jokes. I am having fun.

My Behaviour – I am compiling a joke book and have a leading role in a play.

These examples demonstrate the three elements of our self-concepts. Parents need to be aware of these elements because it is not only what a child "believes" he is but how he feels about himself that determines what he does, i.e., his behaviour. If we are not sensitive to the feeling but merely focus on the beliefs and facts, we will have difficulty changing or improving the self-concept. Facts and beliefs are transient. Feelings are more lasting and difficult to change. In the context of social self-concept above, you may succeed in convincing Sally that she is interesting, that people really don't ignore her, and that she is socially very presentable and a desirable friend (that these are the facts), but if you have not listened to and tried to help her with her gut feelings of anxiety, fear, and self-consciousness, her behaviour, her experimenting with social situations, may not change. Our learned emotions are powerful: they are the fuel for our behaviour and often override hard fact. And they take longer to change. Empathy, acceptance of these feelings, encouragement, modelling, and small stages of growth are required to achieve a change in a desired behaviour.

THE REAL SELF, THE IDEAL SELF, AND THE MASQUERADE SELF

The *real self* refers to how we consciously perceive ourselves to be. This is our honest evauation of what we *believe* we are and how we *feel* about ourselves.

The *ideal self* is the kind of person we would like to be. The ideal self may be beyond reason and beyond reach or may be just a little better than our real self. The difference between the two can be tremendously motivating or devastating. The ideal self is often based on parents' expectations and on their high self-esteem. High expectation, if realistic, can be a positive influence in a child's life. However, if the gap between the real and the ideal is too wide, it can contribute to low self-esteem, to insecurity, to personal devaluation, and to deception.

The deception comes in the form of a *masquerade self*, a set of behavioural masks assumed to portray ourselves as we would like people to think we are. Usually it does not come off too easily. Energies and preoccupation are devoted to "looking good" instead of having the security of being your real self and growing up slowly to the ideal self. If people approve of your masquerade self, your phony front, there is also a dilemma: you then think they only like the counterfeit, which is not really you. Another dilemma is created when the phoniness appeals to people you do not want to impress and the people you want to impress see through the deception.

Since parents are the most powerful influences in the development of a child's self-concept, their expectations are often responsible for the child's need to use a masquerade self in order to please and be accepted. Since much of our self-concept is formed in early and middle childhood and becomes stable for our lifetime, this childhood masquerade sets the stage for a lifetime of deception and insecurity. A major problem in this acting is that often the individual may lose touch with the real self – it has been submerged. The facade, the masquerade self, takes over, but it generally doesn't work because the real self eats away at the insides, festers, and then erupts in some form of physical or psychological sickness.

Society most often sets our values and standards of what is correct, what we should want, what we should be, rather than allowing us to be what we are. Popularity, approval, material and occupational success, and rigidly defined roles are values enshrined in our society that parents translate to children. If parents don't consider whether the roles and expectations fit their particular offspring, there can be damage. As Sid Jourard states, "If a person carries out his roles suitably he can be regarded as a normal personality. Normal personalities, however, are not necessarily healthy personalities." He goes on to say that the pursuit of role conformity can produce anxiety, guilt, boredom, frustration, fatigue, and physical illness. "They sicken because they behave in sickening ways."

THE MASQUERADE IS OVER: THE CASE OF GINNY P.

The following story of Ginny, age seventeen, is the story of a conflict between her two selves – the real self and her masquerade self. No one would have predicted Ginny's breakdown. She had everything – the admiration of parents, friends, a beautiful face, an attractive body, and a great mind. She was her school's top athlete, top scholar, top everything including the Prom Queen. She always seemed to radiate happiness, self-confidence, and boundless energy. Her collapse was sudden and major. Her parents felt the breakdown must have been caused by physical fatigue. It couldn't be psychological, not this happy, terrific-at-everything person. What they didn't know was that the self that showed did not mirror the insecure, frightened self inside. The real self was in agony and conflict with her masquerade self and it never surfaced. Because of her parents', teachers', and everyone's expectation and portrait of Ginny there was no room for failure, for tears, or for her anxieties.

In the quiet of her room she cried and wanted to be a little girl again in the security of her mother's arms. She agonized that people only liked her pretty face, her pretend self; they were not interested in her real or inside self. She felt they wouldn't like her for her insecurities, her unsureness, her fears. It took so much energy to cover up and she never let this inner self surface. The conflict between her two images, the real and what she considered her cosmetic image, generated horrendous pressures and tension. Because she couldn't release this pressure or share it for fear of being exposed, it burst and she was sick. Her sickness was a protest, an escape.

According to Sid Jourard, "when a person behaves in a way that does violence to their integrity, fuses blow, the power is shut off. The meaning of sickness is protest ... being sick is a behaviour to restore integrity." Ginny had become self-alienated; her outside did not reflect her inside self. How amazing it is that parents, who are supposedly so close, do not pick up these "help me" messages. How could Ginny's parents have missed all the signals of her pain? Perhaps Ginny excelled also at her masks and the hiding of her insecurities.

Things are seldom what they seem
Skim milk masquerades as cream
Externals don't portray insides
Jekylls may be masking Hydes
–*Sidney M. Jourard (1971)*

WHAT IS THE BASIS FOR GOOD SELF-ESTEEM?

Stanley Coopersmith is one of the major contributors to our knowledge of the development of a child's self-esteem. For eight years he studied the antecedents and consequences of self-esteem, specifically the effects of the background, personality, and parental treatment of children with high, low, medium, and defensive self-esteem. His bottom line is that a person's self-worth is primarily based on *parental warmth, clearly defined limits,* and *respectful treatment.*

According to Coopersmith, the four indicators of our self-esteem are: (1) how competent we are in our performance of our tasks, i.e., how successful we have been; (2) how well we meet our ethical and moral standards; (3) how much power and control we have over the circumstances that affect us and the control we have over ourselves, i.e., our self-control; and most important, (4) how loved and how accepted we are by our parents.

THE CRITICAL AGENTS IN OUR SELF-ESTEEM

In the early years, children are completely dependent on their parents for their physical needs, safety needs, love needs, and emotional needs, and certainly are dependent on their parents as well for training, teaching, socialization, and feedback as to "who am I?" and "how am I doing?"

The parent is the most influential agent in the development of a child's self-esteem. Parental values, their example, their personality, and their behaviour to a great extent determine whether a child ends up with a high or low self-esteem, which in turn affects the child's successes and failures in life and his or her emotional stability.

95

The messages begin very early in infancy. Our cuddling and gentle caresses, the tone and warmth of our voice, our laughter, our songs, our ease, and our eyes give messages of security, of love, and of acceptance. These are the foundation for the development of a child's self-concept. The development of a child's self-esteem and his behaviour is illustrated in Figures 9-11.

These diagrams, opposite, describe the process that begins with the parent's behaviour toward the child. This behaviour affects the child's belief and feelings about his self-worth, which in turn affects the child's behaviour. The child's behaviour then confirms the parent's opinion of the child. Figure 10 shows the consequences of negative parent behaviour and Figure 11 shows the consequences of positive parent behaviour.

Coopersmith's extensive research gives us important direction as to the parental characteristics and behaviour that affect the development of a child's self-esteem. But before reporting on these patterns of parental characteristics and behaviour, let us see what the pictures are of individuals with high and low self-esteem. Our self-esteem, remember, is defined as our judgement of the worthiness of our values, behaviour, attitudes, and personality.

High Self-esteem Individuals: A Portrait

1. They approach tasks with expectation they will succeed.
2. They approach persons with expectation they will be well-received.
3. They accept their own opinions and judgements and follow their judgements.
4. They trust their reactions and conclusions.
5. They are socially comfortable, show ease in forming and maintaining friendships.
6. They are assertive.
7. They are creative.
8. They are good problem-solvers.
9. They are high achievers and action-oriented.
10. Their lack of preoccupation with personal problems allows them to focus on relevant tasks.
11. They are not self-conscious.
12. They are active participants in discussions rather than listeners.
13. They can be independent and interdependent.
14. They enjoy their family.
15. They respect their parents.
16. They contribute to society.

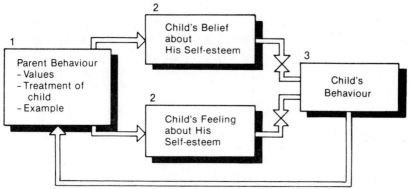

Figure 9. Development of Self-esteem and Behaviour

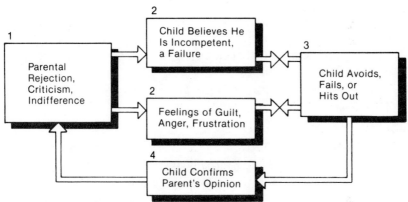

Figure 10. Low Self-esteem Development

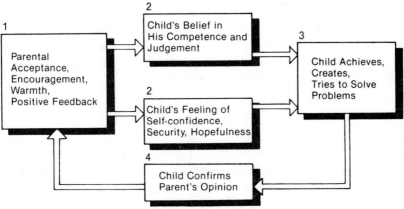

Figure 11. High Self-esteem Development

17. They feel secure.

18. They are aware of their feelings of anger and fear, do not repress them, and can ask for assistance to help resolve them.

19. They know that there will always be problems but have confidence in their skills to cope with them.

20. They are succcessful personally, socially, vocationally, and familialy.

Low Self-esteem Individuals: A Portrait

1. They have difficulties in academic, social, and physical situations.

2. They have feelings of anxiety, insecurity, embarrassment, guilt, and fear.

3. They withdraw from social situations.

4. They lack trust in themselves.

5. They will not attempt anything new.

6. They are self-conscious.

7. They are preoccupied with their feelings and do not focus on the task or the present problem.

8. They are suspicious, distrustful, and envious.

9. They have psychosomatic illnesses.

10. They are dependent.

11. They reject family and friends.

12. They can be physically and verbally aggressive.

13. They put on false fronts to mask their low esteem.

14. They use a number of defense mechanisms to protect themselves, e.g., denial, rationalization, regression, etc.

15. They believe that they do not have control over their lives and their futures or over themselves.

Clearly, people with low self-esteem differ considerably from those with high self-esteem. As might be expected, the parents also differ in their behaviours, demands, and values. The following profiles show just how different the two groups of parents are.

Parents of Children with High Self-esteem

1. Parents of children with a high self-esteem also have a high self-esteem, i.e., they like who they are and value their own opinions and accomplishments. They feel good about themselves and are self-assured. They are on good terms with each other, value their relationships, and have established a good contract between themselves with clear lines of authority and responsibility. They are both very active outside the family and don't have to depend on their family as the only source of gratification.

2. The children are accepted by their parents: I accept you as you are; you're okay and I really like who you are!

3. Parents show concern for the child's welfare: they show respect, affection, support, and attentiveness.

4. They have definite values and clear concepts of what is appropriate and inappropriate behaviour and are prepared to enforce these values and concepts with explanation but without hesitation.

5. Children with high self-esteem have parents who set clear, definite limits, which are enforced with consistency but not harshly or punitively. Within these limits they permit relatively great freedom to their children. In his research Coopersmith found that limits have a facilitating effect by giving children a basis for evaluating their performance. The standards and cues are clear and a child can judge for himself whether he has attained a desired goal. Where limits and goals are ambiguous and fuzzy, someone else has to decode the cues and boundaries. Home limits teach the child how to adjust to the limits of school and society. The importance of setting limits for behaviour is that it gives a child information about the expectations and norms of a group and develops techniques of coping with the outside real world. Coopersmith found that children from homes with definite limits were more likely to be socially acceptable and more capable of dealing with criticism, more independent, and more creative. Clear limits by themselves are not sufficient without parental warmth and acceptance, however; there has to be a blend of these conditions to produce self-esteem.

6. Children who develop a high self-esteem for themselves have parents who expect their children to strive and comply with the high standards they establish. The parents have a high set of expectations for themselves and have achieved a high self-esteem. Their expectations are reality-based, i.e., based on the child's past performance and abilities. For the child these expectations say, "I believe in your ability to succeed." It's a vote of confidence, of encouragement, of support. Perhaps what most children need is direction, a goal and assistance with a plan to reach that goal. These parents transmit from their personal history and convictions that a person can make things happen for himself or herself and that one can be in control of one's destiny. They transmit their confidence to their children. Children with high self-esteem have learned to solve problems with expectation that they will succeed. They don't waste valuable energy on preoccupations with "Will I succeed? What if I fail?" Their preoccupation and energy is concentrated on the task and this increases the probability of their success.

Parents of Children with Low Self-esteem

1. The parents have a low self-esteem of themselves.
2. They have few expectations for their children or themselves.

3. They have a belief that "Nothing I do makes a difference; I have no control over my life." They expect failure.

4. They are distant, inattentive, and neglectful.

5. They don't convey feelings of love, acceptance, or respect.

6. They are punitive, critical, and sarcastic.

7. There are no clear guidelines or limits.

8. Their attitudes create similar attitudes in their children, who anticipate failure and rejection. Some become pensive and withdrawn, others defend their inadequacies and low self-esteem by hitting out aggressively against self, family, or society. The parents are so preoccupied with failure and their negative feelings that they fail to focus on or have the energies for the demands of any task.

Another notable difference between the highs and lows is the difference in the amount of stimulation: the homes of the high self-esteem children provide an environment with a high level of activity, planning, doing, verbal exchange, and opportunities for listening and sharing in one-to-one situations.

Most parents, to be sure, don't fit neatly into one category or the other. Most of us fit somewhere in between. The value of Coopersmith's research is that it gives us the explanations and guidelines for improvement. Children are not the only ones in need of models. The characteristics and behaviour of the parents of the high self-esteem children give us a direction and goals to emulate. When parents stop growing, when they stop trying to improve, when they feel that there is nothing left to learn or that it is too late to learn, they and their children may be in for trouble. What is important to remember is that differences reflect a pattern of conditions and that for high self-esteem to develop we must ask these questions:

- As a parent, what is your self-esteem?
- Is your marriage in good shape?
- Have you defined specific clear limits and enforced them?
- Have you defined specific freedoms and responsibilities?
- Do you have high but reasonable expectations with demonstration of support, encouragement, and example?
- Do you show your love, your complete acceptance, and your regard for your children?
- Are you just preoccupied with your children or do you have other means of gratification?
- Is your home stimulating?
- Do you have one-to-one times to listen and to share?

If you can answer these questions positively, then the climate is there for the development of a healthy self-concept in your children.

OTHER INFLUENCES

There are many other influences and agents in the development of a self-concept in children in addition to parents. These include sisters, brothers, grandparents, relatives, friends, teachers, the media, and the society we live in. Next to parents, the most powerful agent is the school system and, specifically, a child's teacher. Stars, marks, grades, teacher's comments, and school privileges vividly and sometimes painfully give us information about who we are and how we are doing. Our self-concept is built on this feedback. Our concept of smartness and dumbness is fashioned and sometimes warped by these messages. Often they reflect only a present ability and not the capacity or potential, but they can put a lid on this potential. "I don't know how to read, I get unsatisfactories, my teacher is unhappy with me, my parents are unhappy with me, my friends tease me, I feel anxious, ashamed, and I really don't like myself. I'm a dummy, and my marks tell me so." This low self-concept becomes the precursor for future failure and self-fulfilling prophecies.

PROGNOSIS FOR GROWTH OR REPAIR

There are no magic pills to change or repair a poor self-concept. Though a person's self-concept begins to take shape very early in childhood (about the age of five) and becomes quite fixed and stable between the ages of twelve to eighteen, there are ways to assist in the change and improvement of a child's or adolescent's self-image.

Change begins with an understanding of the anatomy and complexity of the self-concept, including that:

- a self-concept is made up of three basic elements, a set of beliefs, of behaviours, and of feelings;
- we have a number of sub-self-concepts, e.g., the physical, moral-ethical, social, personal, and school or work self-concepts;
- there are three selves, the real self, the ideal self, and the masquerade self;
- parents' behaviour and values and child-rearing styles affect it;
- school, peers, and society also affect the development of self-esteem; and
- a self-concept is an evaluation of our successes and failures, an evaluation of how we perceive that others value and accept us, and an evaluation of how we cope with criticism and devaluation.

Figure 12 suggests the circular process of high and low self-esteem. The question is how do you break into this process?

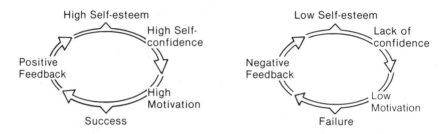

Figure 12. Circular Process of High and Low Self-esteem

Steps to be taken to break the tight circle of low self-esteem should include the following recommendations.

1. Take an inventory of what you perceive your child's self-concept to be and what your child perceives it to be – what he likes about himself, what he dislikes, and what he would like to change.

2. Get to know not only his beliefs about all his sub-selves but "listen for the feeling" about himself. Begin this process by (a) sharing something of yourself with him, which gives him licence and an invitation to share himself with you. Share your thoughts, your own expectations, your ambitions, your failures, and your successes; (b) be empathetic, i.e., for a moment in time try to imagine and feel what he feels, what it must be like to be him, perhaps his loneliness or lack of confidence; (c) don't judge, but listen and give him a message that you love and accept him as he is; and (d) create an atmosphere so that he can move, experiment, and even fail without fear or without a need for a facade or defence.

3. Help him define his problems and help him with his alternatives to solve these problems. An important way of doing this is by modelling, i.e., by the example of your behaviour, how you resolve problems and ambiguities, how you make decisions, how you deal with failure and success.

4. Be aware of his expectations and declare your expectations. They give him a note of confidence, direction, and a plan. But since his self-esteem is low, break down these expectations into small digestible chunks so that he can succeed. When he succeeds (see Figure 12) he will get positive feedback from you and others, which leads to greater self-esteem, self-confidence, motivation, and success.

5. Set up clear limits and guidelines that give him boundaries and standards for what is acceptable and unacceptable. The vagueness of limits is not freedom, for ambiguities cause insecurities. He needs specific guidelines and limits with built-in freedoms within the limits and an

opportunity to expand these limits on the basis of performance.

Finally, if there is a set of conditions in the home that includes love, regard, acceptance, humour, positive stimulation, and activity, a climate that encourages exploration and sees failure or mistakes as part of the learning process and where feelings can surface and be acceptable, then the likelihood that a self-concept is being stepped on is minimal.

SEVEN

Contracts and Conflicts

The happiness, prosperity and strength of a society begins with the adherence to family rules.
— DEUTERONOMY

A major source of generation conflict lies in a real or imagined violation of implicit contractual agreements.
— DAVID ELKIND (1979)

Every human relationship and encounter involves a contract, an understanding, an agreement, a set of rules.

Man is by nature a rule-forming, rule-following, and rule-violating creature.

The essence of this chapter is the thesis that a contract exists in all families and that if conflict occurs it is because of a bad contract. A contract is defined as an understanding, an agreement, a set of expectations, rules, and responsibilities. A clear parent-child contract is needed because the family is a complex, multifaceted institution with many needs and many functions. It must have a well-defined organizational structure to actualize disparate goals as the satisfying of physical, intellectual, educational, emotional, social, and economic needs.

If a parent-child or family contract is to be effective, it must include the following elements: clarity, explicitness, open and regular communications, rules, responsibilities, consequences, procedures for discussion, ventilation, renegotiation, and evaluation. It must reflect the philosophy, expectations, and needs of all members of the family and be capable of adjusting to the dynamic changes of age and stage. Above all, it must be based on faith, mutual respect, and a loving attitude.

Strangers, Antagonists, and Bad Contracts

It often occurs to me as I sit in consultation with parents and children who are in the midst of conflict that I sit with strangers. They don't know each other and have never communicated with each other. They begin to hear expectations, needs, feelings, and complaints as if for the first time.

Other times, I feel as if I sit in an arena of warring antagonists and arch competitors where one side must win and one side must lose, and where there is too much heat but little light. I am asked to be the arbitrator or referee or judge. Often, since the parent is more powerful and is paying for the consultation, I am expected to support the more powerful antagonist.

As I sit and listen and listen I begin to feel as if I am watching a rerun of a rerun of an old problem. The problem is generally not a lack of love, caring, or good intent. It is more often a problem of a bad contract.

WHAT IS A CONTRACT?

Every human grouping and interaction, be it two people, four, or a thousand, operates with some expectations, rules, understanding, and responsibilities, and with some consequences. This, essentially, is a contract. There are good contracts and bad contracts, clear contracts, fuzzy contracts, fair contracts, unspoken contracts, unreasonable, exploitative, and burdensome contracts. There are contracts or understandings between husband and wife, parent and child, teacher and pupil, citizens and government. Even a casual meeting in an elevator where someone you don't know says, "Good morning, can I press your floor for you?" constitutes a contract. There is an implicit understanding and an expectation that you in return will respond with a "Good morning, forty-four please. Thank you." This is a simple contract between two strangers.

A contract between teacher and pupil is more complex. Some of the provisions in this contract include an expectation that the teacher is trained, knows her subject, can teach, explains her classroom rules, is sensitive to individual differences, can motivate, is a good model, likes children, and is excited about education. A teacher's expectation of the student includes his or her being on time, rested, motivated, attentive, interested, obedient, skilled in the prerequisites for the subject, completing assignments, asking questions, and learning the material.

WHY A PARENT-CHILD OR FAMILY CONTRACT?

"Contracts are for strangers!" "A family doesn't need a contract. It sounds too legal!"

Unfortunately the word "contract" has developed formal and legalistic overtones. As stated above, our definition of contract is an agreement, a set of expectations, an understanding of give and take, rules, responsibilities, and consequences. A contract exists in a good or bad form in every family even though it may not necessarily be written out, signed, witnessed, or agreed to by all members of the family.

No other personal relationship is so close, physically and emotionally, for so long as a parent-child relationship. The intensity and duration and differences in needs and age make it easy for problems and conflicts to develop which can affect the mental and physical health of both parent and child.

Running a home, bringing up a family, is not a simple task. A family is a complex, demanding organization and like many other organizations, social, professional, governmental, educational, or economic, there must be clearly defined goals, rights, rules, and responsibilities for it to run effectively and for the good of all.

As a parent in our society, you are expected to provide and administrate for your children food, clothing, shelter, safety and health needs, love, affection, and encouragement. You are expected to educate, to socialize, and to be a model for your child. In turn, we have a long list of real and unreal expectations for our children including being responsible, committed, loyal, and a source of positive feedback. Specifically, we expect them to participate in the chores of the household, learn and conform to the rules of the family and society, be good at school, be popular, enjoy their friends, respect our privacy and possessions, love, honour, and obey us and ignore parental inconsistencies, develop good health and social habits, play the piano, etc., etc., etc.

How well do all these expectations fit together? How do you actualize all these goals and expectations without chaos, confusion, conflict? What is the organizational structure? What expertise is needed and what rules? For all these things to happen in a harmonious environment, it is critical to have a good parent-child contract. The following everyday conflict situations underline the need for a clear contract:

"If I bring home my friends, you complain; if I go out to see them, you complain. I can't win!"

"You can't use the car anymore. Using the car is a privilege and includes cleaning out the coke bottles, the ash trays, and the lipstick on the upholstery and returning it with gas."

"Who was on the phone for the past four hours?"

"I heard you quit school last month. Why?"

"How can you tell him not to smoke if you smoke two packs a day?"

"You expect me to clean the house, be on the gymnastic team, get good grades, and work on Saturday. That's child abuse!"

"Mom chews gum, why can't I?"

"Did God create boys to be allergic to dishwashing?"

"You want me to read; comic books is reading. What was the last book you read, Dad?"

"I heard you were caught drinking at school and expelled. Why didn't you tell me?"

Parent-Child Contracts

BASIC CLAUSES

How would a contract eliminate these problems and conflicts? What are the clauses, the agreements, the elements of a good parent-child contract? What are the procedures for developing a contract? Professor Elkind of Tufts University, who has studied parent-child conflicts and their effects, suggests that conflicts are not unhealthy, that they are part of the process of growth to maturity. He differentiates three types of arrangements between parents and children that are used to resolve the inevitable conflicts. These arrangements include a bargain, an agreement, and a contract.

A BARGAIN

A bargain is the simplest of all arrangements between parent and child. In a bargain a parent offers specific rewards or punishment for specific behaviours. One example of a bargain in early childhood might be: "You can have the car tonight if you wash it this weekend." Bargains can also be initiated by the child or adolescent, e.g., "I'll polish your car for $10."

AN AGREEMENT

An agreement is a more elaborate bargain where both parents and child agree to comply with specific rules over an indefinite period. There may be an agreement that an adolescent's room is out of bounds to his six-year-old sister; that children must knock before entering their parents' bedroom; that Dad gets to read the evening paper before Jan and Jon begin cutting it up for a school project; or that "you don't have to eat a new food, but you do have to try it."

According to Professor Elkind three basic clauses to a contract exist in every one of the major growth periods – infancy, preschool, middle childhood, and adolescence. They are: the responsibility-freedom clause, the achievement-support clause, and the loyalty-commitment clause.

1. *The responsibility-freedom clause* includes parental expectations that certain personal and household responsibilities and duties will be assumed in return for certain freedoms, autonomy, and privileges.

2. *The achievement-support clause* relates to both the parents' and child's expectations for psychological support and for encouragement toward achievement. The support following successful performance includes both psychological and material support.

3. *The loyalty-commitment clause* deals with the expectations that, though there are changes in both parent and child needs, they each remain committed to the other to take care of these needs and they maintain their emotional bonds and ties.

Although these three clauses of parent-child contracts clearly describe the essence of the parent-child expectations, the danger is that most expectations are *implicit* rather than *explicit*. There are just too many assumptions: "I didn't know you expected me to earn my own money for books?" Or, "Why didn't you tell me that it was important to you that I go to your shcool play and to your swim meet? I just assumed I would only make you nervous." These conflicts and grievances develop, simmer, and erupt because a contract needs more than expectations; it needs form, structure, and procedures.

To eliminate the "shooting from the hip" or "accusations on the run" situations that include charges, recriminations, and defensiveness, a family has to have a set of procedures that include a specific time and place for the airing of complaints and expectations and for discussion and resolution of differences. To the objection that "we don't have time for such meetings" I suggest that usually more time, energy, and preoccupation is spent on accusations and defence than on planning and on the strategies and procedures to resolve differences.

The Basic Elements of a Good Contract

From in-depth analysis of families who are in constant conflict and from analysis of families where parents and children genuinely enjoy the experience of living together, the elements, the ingredients, and the mechanics for good contracting become obvious. A contract should attend to the following questions:

1. Is the contract clear?
2. Is it explicit?
3. Does it reflect the philosophy, needs, and expectations of *all* partners?
4. Is it sensitive to ages and stages (intellectual, emotional, social, and physical) of development?
5. What are the specific rules?
6. What are the responsibilities?
7. What are the privileges and freedoms?
8. What are the specific consequences of a breach of the contract?
9. What are the consequences of adherence to the contract?
10. Is the contract fair?
11. Is it dynamic and flexible?
12. Is there good communication?
13. What is the level of commitment?
14. What is the duration of the contract?
15. What are the procedures for the following?
    (a) ventilation of complaints
    (b) resolution of conflicts
    (c) evaluation of the contract
    (d) renegotiation of the contract
16. Does the contract reflect empathy, faith, and respect?
17. When are family meetings held? Where? Who conducts the meeting? What are the rules of the meeting?

Consideration of these elements gives the contract structure, direction, a plan, a feeling, and helps to create a positive environment where parents can manage, grow, and enjoy parenting and where a child can grow and develop in a warm, secure climate.

CLARITY, EXPLICITNESS, AND COMMUNICATION

Is the understanding clear and explicit? Too many expectations are implied, too many understandings are assumed. State your contract in language that all members of the family can understand. Sometimes clarity needs time and repetition. Don't assume that others hear or perceive as you do. Check their perceptions as they should check yours. Give your children the time and the privilege to state their understanding or expectations in their own style and manner. The experience they develop in family contracts will be invaluable in the contracts they will be involved with as they grow up and out.

A contract must be a reflection of the philosophy, values, needs, and goals of all parties in the contract. Prior to the development of a parent-child contract, it is important and realistic that the parents establish a harmonious contract between themselves to deal with their expectations of each other, their values, needs, and motives. A husband-wife contract that attends to all the elements is the basic foundation and the model for the parent-child contract.

Both parents and children have needs, expectations, and rights that should be taken into account in formulating a contract. For children these might include:

- love, maintenance, protection, and education
- parental time
- parental understanding of the stages of child development
- parenting skills
- reasonable limits
- regular schedules
- praise and reinforcement
- fully attentive listening
- empathetic listening
- someone to hold on to and let go of
- somone to ask countless questions, to clarify thinking
- opportunities to explore
- opportunities to make mistakes and learn from these mistakes without being threatened by a sense of failure
- opportunities to share a fantasy
- opportunities to learn rules and practise rules
- opportunities to develop rules
- privacy
- acceptance in the experiencing of ambivalent emotions of love and hate, approach and avoidance
- a peer group
- enhancement of self-esteem
- the sense of belonging
- someone to imitate and model
- responsibility and freedom
- the opportunity to excel at something
- the opportunity to develop according to one's own maturational timetable

- freedom to own one's own problems
- good one-to-one relationships with members of the family

Parents, of course, also have rights and expectations that need to be fulfilled. They must be seen and must see themselves as more than the caterers to their children's every whim. Their needs and rights might include:

- education and training for parenthood
- assistance from spouse
- children who share responsibilities and observe family rules
- children who listen and try to understand
- love, warmth, and feedback from their children
- professional assistance with the problems of physical and mental growth
- time for themselves – privacy
- relief from some of the "burdensome pressures" in parenting such as the sameness and routine of feeding, chauffeuring, etc.
- freedom to make mistakes and be forgiven
- opportunities to share their concerns and problems
- time to further individual interests
- assistance with the duties of a household
- expectations related to achievement in social, religious, athletic, and moral behaviour

It should be noted that these lists of children's and parents' needs and expectations, which should be taken into account in the formulation of a contract, only exemplify some of the more basic needs and rights and are not meant to be all-inclusive.

SENSITIVITY TO STAGE AND AGE OF CHILD

Parent-child contracts and arrangements should recognize the age, stage, and abilities of a child and not overwhelm or take advantage of the child's immaturity. They proceed from the simple, temporary bargain at the preschool levels to the more complex, long-term contract in middle childhood and adolescence. Whether they are simple or complex they should, at all stages, be sensitive to and include the elements of a good contract.

Erik Erikson's stages of child and adolescent development and the psychosocial crises typical of each age suggest important guidelines in the development of a parent-child contract. Erikson categorizes the growth and development of children in five stages.

Stage 1: Trust vs. Mistrust, 0-2 years of age. In this stage children are developing a sense of trust as opposed to mistrust. The contract has to include consistent, predictable, care-giving procedures of feeding, cuddling, gentling, speaking to, singing, and changing. The child begins to trust his environment, which is primarily his mother. Erikson believes that at this stage there is a contract of getting and giving. An infant gets the basic care it needs and gives the parent emotional gratification in return.

Stage 2: Autonomy vs. Shame and Doubt, 2-3 years of age. The "terrible twos" need very special contract provisions that allow them "to hold on and to let go." The contract has to allow for the child's clumsy attempt at independent function – "No! I want to feed myself" – even though there is more Jello on the floor than in his mouth. Where the original contract was total dependency and total responsibility, Mother (and Father) has to change the terms and allow for this messy and sometimes inept transition.

Stage 3: Initiatives vs. Guilt, 3-6 years of age. A child can develop a sense of guilt if he or she is reprimanded or punished for attempts at initiative. At this stage children must try out and explore new physical and social roles. A good contract recognizes these needs, reinforces initiative behaviours that are acceptable, and helps a child recognize the consequences of unacceptable behaviours.

Stage 4: Industry vs. Inferiority, 6-12 years of age. The major theme in middle childhood is the motivation to master not only things but social relationships. The conflict here is not being good enough. There is a desire to be first or best. Play activities and personal feelings at this stage reflect competition rather than co-operation. If parents are aware of this internal conflict and tension in the child it helps them in establishing their expectations and their contract. If the contract expects too much, there is a sense of failure and the development of a sense of inferiority.

Stage 5: Identity vs. Role Confusion, 12-18 years of age. This stage includes the crises of puberty and adolescence. The child's overriding question is, "Who am I?" There is a sense of role confusion, of ambivalent love-hate attitudes and feelings toward parents. The parents are replaced by peer group models and standards and the peer group becomes a chief agent of support. But a need still exists for some attachment. The wish for financial independence, coupled with the fact of financial dependence, creates great confusion and the contract has to be supersensitive to this most difficult of all growth crises. A new partnership has to be developed that allows for freedom, error, and initiative yet includes responsibility.

Parents also go through stages and crises. They need their children for different reasons at different ages. For so many years parents are geographically, physically, and emotionally close and involved with their children and then there is a need by children for distance. This distance can be a comfortable distance with mutual support or a break-out distance. Erikson points out that crises are not necessarily bad, since they are needed for growth and development. The value of Erikson's notion of stages of development is that it gives us some understanding of what we can expect from our children as they mature.

FAIRNESS

A contract should be fair, which does *not* mean equal. The age and stage of children dictate their needs, and reasonable privileges, freedoms, and responsibilities. What would be a fair contract for a seven-year-old is not a fair contract for a twelve-year-old. Bedtimes, allowances, and house-hold chores should be age-related.

A contract is not made for ever. Contracts should not be rigid; they should be sensitive to changes of resources, circumstances, interests, health, condition, age, and individual needs. A contract should have built-in mechanisms or procedures to sense changes in needs and to be able to adjust to them.

RULES, LIMITS, AND CONSEQUENCES OF BREACH

Rules should be clear and explicit and should serve a useful function – we do not need rules for rules' sake. They should serve the family as a whole and be consistent. Limits and rules give children stability and facilitate their development. Parents should not be exempt from rules nor from the consequences of breach of rules. They serve as models and their behaviour in reference to rules sets the standard for children to imitate. Consequences should be fair, consistent, and immediate and should only attend to the rule-breaking behaviour and not to past history. The consequence should deal specifically with the rule-breaking behaviour in such a way as not to insult, damage, or reproach a child's self-esteem.

PROCEDURES FOR VENTILATION, EVALUATION,
AND RENEGOTIATION

These elements of a contract are critical. There must be a specific time, a specific place, a specific procedure for someone who is upset with the contractual arrangements to be able to share them with an empathetic family or a specific member of the family. If this expression is encouraged and allowed it will prevent emotional flare-ups, arguments, ill feelings, jealousies, and conflicts from developing. It's often too late if there is no safety valve for the *ventilation* of a complaint or suggestion.

A parent-child contract should be *evaluated* at specific times in terms of its effectiveness, its clarity, its explicitness, its sensitivity to age, needs, and expectations, and its ability to resolve differences. Are the rules and responsibilities fair and are they working? Is the contract creating a harmonious environment where all members of the family are able to develop their abilities and interests, enjoy and support each other, and enjoy being part of the family unit? Following an evaluation of the effectiveness of the contract there should be an opportunity and procedure to *renegotiate* the contract.

These are the essential elements. They must be moulded and formed so that they reflect the needs, circumstances, and personality of your family. The specifics, e.g., the rules, the responsibilities, the when, how, and where you meet to plan and discuss your contract should fit your own family style.

I have been concerned with the consequences of parents slavishly following parenting recipes. They often result in frustration and questions of why the recipe didn't work. Children are sensitive and often recognize and react to the imposition of a "canned parenting procedure." For example, some parenting recipes for communication between parent and child suggest that the parent repeat back to the child what the parent perceives the child is saying for verification purposes. The recipe suggests a specific procedure but the following conversation illustrates, perhaps facetiously, what might happen:

CHILD: I hate my sisters!
PARENT: You really don't like them.
CHILD: I just said that! Are you reading that book again? You sound silly.
PARENT: I really must sound silly.
CHILD: I think I'll burn that book!
PARENT: You do and I'll burn your bottom!

In this case the parent parroted the procedure rather than adapting its essence, which is to let your child know that you are really trying to understand what he is saying without prejudgements.

Purposes, Structure, and Procedure of Family Meetings

Having expressed my concern for the mechanical replication of a suggestion or procedure, I offer the following only as guidelines for family meetings to develop your own individual contract.

Family meetings are held to establish and to monitor the family contract. A family meeting is a multi-purpose vehicle which should serve (1) to define clearly each individual's role in the family; (2) to act as a forum for expectations; (3) for the explanation of rules and the consequences of breach or adherence to the rules; (4) for the discussion and planning of fair workloads and duties; (5) to plan family projects, family trips, vacations, and new acquisitions; (6) to report the sad, the funny, the failures, and the successes; (7) to air complaints or concerns and to resolve conflicts in an atmosphere where the focus is on resolution, not blaming; (8) as a training ground for children to learn how to organize and express their thoughts; (9) for parents and children to learn how to listen attentively to each other with empathy; (10) to give each member of the family a sense of belonging, a sense of safety, security, and status; and (11) to integrate, to involve, and to coalesce all the members of the family in a harmonious, loving environment.

Do you need meetings to actualize these purposes? From the examination of families in conflict I have come to the conclusion that they are necessary for the development of a good contract and for the implementation of that contract. The family is a complex organization and each member's needs can best be satisfied with planning and communication. A contract is the plan; a meeting is the communication.

In every family there are a number of contracts. There is a contract (good or bad) between husband and wife, between each parent and each child, between one child and another; and there is the family contract. How productive are the family contract and almost all other contracts generally depends on the contract, the style, and the morale that exist between the parents. As in any organization, morale begins at the top and it affects and infects all levels of the organization. If mother and father are at war, the family meetings will be battles, not councils of peace and harmony. Parents have to get their act together first.

STRUCTURE AND PROCEDURE

Meetings should be held at least once a month at a specific place and a specific time. Everyone should attend. To begin, a parent should act as the chairperson of the meeting until one of the children can assume that role. At that point a system of revolving responsibility for the position can be established.

The meeting should have a specific agenda made up of issues and suggestions supplied by members of the family. Every member must be made aware of the agenda prior to the meeting and must have sufficient time to express his or her views.

As most of us are aware, even meetings between relatively homogeneous adults can be difficult to conduct. Because of the difference in ages or the difference in understanding, in needs, and in expressive ability, the chairperson must exercise great judgement and sensitivity. Learning how to conduct enjoyable and productive sessions follows the Learning-Hope Curve (see p. 59). At first the meetings may not be very satisfactory, but with time they get better. If the goal of the meeting is to develop a forum for the family to conduct its affairs for the good of all and not as a forum to arbitrarily hand out rules and reprimands, Stage 2 of the Learning-Hope Curve will be realized.

THE SOMERVILLE CONTRACT

The Somervilles are a family of five: Bill and Kay Somerville and their three children. Cliff is fifteen years old, Cynthia is thirteen, and Carl is seven. Bill is a buyer for a department store chain and Kay works two and a half days a week as a telephone operator. Cliff is in grade eleven, plays for the school basketball team, works Saturdays on the check-out counter of a supermarket, and has a special girlfriend, Theresa. Cynthia is in grade nine, plays flute in the school orchestra, and has inherited Cliff's paper route. Carl has a severe learning disability, is in a special class, and has difficulty with his motor and language functioning.

Bill and Kay had worked out a good contract between themselves before the children arrived and are still working on it. They began their family meetings when Cliff was about seven. Over the years, Bill and Kay Somerville have demonstrated a great deal of affection and caring for their children. They clearly outlined what their children could expect from them in terms of time, instruction, assistance, and facilities. They also clearly outlined all the duties and responsibilities that were needed to run the household and that every member had to share these duties if it was to operate smoothly. No one would be taken advantage of and no one would get a free ride. Since Mother was working two and a half days and taking a course at night to complete a degree, she needed extra help and lots of co-operation. They looked forward to and thoroughly enjoyed their monthly meetings and would not allow anything to interfere with them. It was a number one priority the first Sunday of every month. Cliff and Cynthia were now taking their turns to chair the meetings. The following is an agenda for one of their Sunday meetings, which covered a range of family and personal issues.

1. Kay Somerville wants to discuss her plans to go back full-time to university for a business degree. There are financial considerations as well as a change in her duties at home.
2. Cynthia would like to discuss a new piano as well as her concerns for her privacy.

3. The garage needs a coat of paint and Dad would like to set a specific time for painting.
4. Aunt Hilda had asked if she could come and visit for the month of June.
5. The family had to decide whether they should rent a summer cottage again since Cliff wanted to work in the city and Cynthia wanted to take a trip to Oregon to visit her grandmother.
6. Carl wanted to talk about a problem at school. Some of the kids were calling him dummy and retardo at recess and on the way home.

It should be noted that at least some of the agenda items, especially the final one, will have been considered prior to the meeting on a one-to-one basis between family members. Not all things are specifically held back just for the family meeting.

In the meeting they presented, they listened, they discussed, they argued, they resolved, and they planned. Sometimes there were tears. Sometimes there was laughter. Sometimes someone said something he/she didn't mean. They had one important rule and that was that a meeting was never adjourned in anger. They believed that their relationship was more important than any one issue and that there was some solution to every issue.

The content of the agenda speaks volumes of where this family is at, what their contract is like, and how important their family meetings are to them. The Somervilles have their share of problems. A good contract and their family meetings do not eliminate their problems, but they help them to focus on and to resolve the difficulties without creating more problems. Cliff, Cynthia, and Carl know what they can expect from their parents and what is expected of them. They live and grow in a warm, secure climate of mutual respect. There are no hidden agendas, since they are encouraged to keep their concerns and conflicts out in the open where they can be dealt with.

Some Final Observations

Because the contract and expectations are clear, explicit, and agreed upon, the focus and energies of the family are directed on productive growth, work, play, and achievement and not on bickering or battle. The realization that contracts exist in all interpersonal relationships – at home, at play, at school, at work, and in all societal encounters – is important for child, adolescent, and parent. Parents who habitually fail to fulfil their contractual obligations are often the cause of their children's anxieties, delinquency, or revolt. On the other hand, the successful parent-child contract becomes the basis for the many subsequent contracts the child will be involved in. Learning the elements, the development, the workings, and the consequences of a good contract at home gives the child the experience, confidence, and skills to participate in future contracts in school, in his job, in organizations, and in his future family. A family contract becomes the model for others. Clear contracts with oneself and others lead to effective self-control.

Present research gives evidence of the effect of good contracts on a child's personality. It has been demonstrated that fair, clear, comprehensive, consistent, and enforced parental rules lead to greater emotional stability and higher self-esteem in children. It is more productive for a parent to look at a specific misbehaviour or conflict in terms of what's wrong with the contract rather than attacking a child's personality; in other words, rearrange the contract, not the child's personality. A contract that considers mutual expectations results in mutual respect.

Finally, a contract of some kind exists in all families. If there is constant conflict, it's a symptom of a bad contract.

EIGHT

Does Discipline Mean Punishment?

18th Century: The Age of the Puritan Ethic

Children are like the Devil with foolish desires and groveling appetites like beasts of the field. Their will must be broken.
— **JOHN WESLEY**

19th Century: The Age of Reason

There is an innate goodness in children and a capacity to reason. These natural virtues need only to be encouraged. There is no real reason to harden children nor to break their will through beating.
— **JEAN JACQUES ROUSSEAU**

20th Century : The Age of Progress?

The human buttocks are admirably designed for character building.
— **CHAPMAN, 1956**

Spanking is simply the most effective...it works. Be careful of tissue damage.
— **KILLORY, 1974**

The majority of the Supreme Court Justices ruled that corporal punishment in school does not violate the 8th Amendment to the U.S. Constitution.
— **NEWS REPORT, 1977**

Harsh punishment inflicted in anger relieves the parent's overcharged mind, but, in most cases, serves no other useful purpose and in the last analysis does irremediable harm. Spanking and whipping are the easiest forms of punishment and the least intelligent.
— **BROWN, 1923**

What is wrong with spanking is the lesson it demonstrates...when you are angry – hit! Instead of displaying our ingenuity by finding civilized outlets for savage feeling we give our children a taste of the jungle.
— **DR. HAIM GINOTT, 1965**

This chapter explores the meaning of discipline and presents the case of Kelly T. to illustrate the problems caused by harsh and inconsistent discipline. Historically, discipline meant to educate; currently it is more often defined as punishment. Goals of discipline are suggested, such as the learning of social judgement, social rules, family rules and responsibilities, and the ultimate goal of self-discipline and self-control.

The four basic methods of discipline, i.e., reward, punishment, rational explanation, and modelling are assessed. Research evidence on the efficacy of different parenting styles and their relationship to the development of self-discipline is reported. This chapter also explores the advantages, disadvantages, and dangers of various forms of punishment.

Thirteen Therapists Later: The Case of Kelly T. (age 15)

MRS. T. You're the thirteenth professional I've seen. I hope you have some answers for me. My husband and daughter absolutely refuse to see another professional.

DR. M.: Thirteenth? That makes me nervous. What's the problem?

MRS. T.: We desperately need some help with Kelly. Perhaps you can suggest where we can send her. Do you know of a good girls' school where she can learn some self-discipline, get a good education, and become something? I've tried everything, you name it and we've tried it. Family therapy, family counselling, transactional analysis, Gestalt, Rational Emotive Therapy, P.E.T., and Reality Therapy. I should be given a degree in psychology but I wouldn't take it – nothing worked.

    I not only tried all the therapies, I've tried changing schools, houses, church, and almost considered changing my husband.

DR. M. Tell me about Kelly.

MRS. T.: Right now she is on probation. She was picked up drunk at a rock concert where she assaulted a policeman. She has run away three times with different men and has had one abortion. It's impossible to control her. She skips school, has failed twice, and is in a constant running battle with her teachers.

    She is having a terrible effect on her two young sisters. We've tried to protect the little ones, but they have already had a terrible fight because her twelve-year-old sister found her diaphragm and told her father, who then gave Kelly a beating. She's going down the drain and I am afraid she's taking the family with her.

DR. M. Tell me what you like about Kelly? What are her strengths?

MRS. T. Her strengths? I guess her body and her good looks.

DR. M. Nothing else?

MRS. T. She's great with her grandparents. She stays with them when they are sick, cooks, washes, and cleans for them. She is really tender and loving with them. When my mother had an operation on her hip, she didn't leave the hospital for two nights. I think she likes them better than us.

She's great with dogs and loves babies. She used to babysit a lot until she was caught having sex with her boyfriend while she was babysitting. It got around and now no one wants to hire her. I think it also might be because a couple of fathers have tried to proposition her.

She's very good at music, but I took her guitar away after the rock concert brawl. She's been a problem since she was three. Sometimes I wish I never had children.

DR. M. How does Kelly feel about her life, about her probation, her abortion, her drinking, her sleeping around?

MRS. T. She's never told me, but I've read her diary. She's miserable – she writes that she hates herself. She feels guilty, dirty, and talks about her Other Self, her wild self that makes her do all these things. She doesn't enjoy drinking and has had only one satisfying sexual experience out of about fifteen. Sometimes she mentioned that she loves me, but most of the time there is hate for me and for her father. She is really frightened when he hits her and threatens to send her to training school. She believes he could and might do it. That diary scares me.

DR. M. What about Mr. T.? How does he feel about Kelly and about what she does? What does he do about it?

MRS. T. He's a blank! The only thing he can do is make a living. He really doesn't get involved with the kids at all unless it's to go to church. He likes his girls all dressed up on Sunday and likes to parade them into church. He's an elder in our church. He's a salesman, travels a lot, drinks a lot, and I think he screws around a lot. He's always "too tired" when he gets home from a sales trip. He's even too tired when he's not on a sales trip. Two years of family therapy didn't help much. I'm working part-time now and I've got a couple of male friends. A person has needs, you know. I've also unfortunately gained twenty pounds from binge eating this past year.

DR. M. What do you and Mr. T. usually do when Kelly or your other two daughters do something that displeases you?

MRS. T. He usually spanks them or threatens them with his belt. I don't believe kids should be hit, certainly not girls, so he and I usually end up having our own fight. He has threatened to send Kelly to a training school.

I've tried everything – love, affection, yelling, taking away privileges, promising them new clothes, jewelry, sending them to their room, but never, never hitting.

DR. M. What responsibilities do Kelly and her sisters have around the house?

MRS. T. Not many. They're only kids. They really have it easy. As long as they hang up their clothes, keep themselves clean, eat properly, and do their homework, that's all I ask. I do the rest. Everything – the meals, the dishes, cleaning, laundry, sewing, shopping, the bills, taking them to their music lessons, the dentist, and doctor.

DR. M. I'm curious; if I'm number thirteen, when did you begin to look for professional assistance?

MRS. T. When Kelly was five she ran away. I took her to see a child psychiatrist for about a year, but that didn't help. I didn't even tell my husband about that one. I've been to school counsellors, psychiatrists, psychologists, social workers, child-care workers, family therapists, and my clergyman. I am beginning to lose faith in professionals.

I love that kid so much and I wish I could help her. Do you know of any residential school I could send her to? I'd sell the house, anything, to help her.

Is sending Kelly away the solution? That seems to be the final alternative for parents. By sending them away they assume that someone else will correct the problem. This often compounds the problem, the pain, and the frustrations for child and family. Thirteen professionals later, Mrs. T. had truly become sophisticated in the professional jargon and techniques. She may well have deserved a degree in psychology, but she had not learned or earned a degree in parenting. Her understanding of a child's needs and her parenting skills had not really improved over the fifteen years. She began with love and affection for Kelly and fifteen years later still loved her deeply, agonized over her pain, and felt totally frustrated. Where had she gone wrong?

As one takes inventory of this sad situation, a number of problems surface. Mr. and Mrs. T. were ill-prepared for parenthood in terms of their attitudes, understanding of growth and development, or any parenting skills. Perhaps even more critical was the bad contract between them. His drinking and carousing, her overeating, their extra-marital sexual indulgences, the absence of any sensitivity to each other's needs and expectations, the lack of rules, and the uneven burden of responsibilities set the scene for what was to follow. They began with poor self-discipline and ended up as poor models for their children. The word "discipline" was a red flag to Mrs. T.; it conjured up physical punishment and child abuse.

She loved her children so much that rules and responsibilities interfered with her notion of loving and giving. The children had no opportunity in the home to learn external limits and control and then to develop their own self-control. Mother did everything for them and took away the necessary and invaluable learning that comes from participation in family responsibilities. There were no limits or guidelines for Kelly to learn; hence she had difficulty coping with family, school, and society.

Kelly desperately needed to be needed. She needed limits, rules, responsibilities, and an opportunity to be party to the development of these rules and responsibilities. Her "Other Self," her "Wild Self," was a product of inconsistent discipline, the mixture of love and physical punishment, of fear, of parental misbehaviour, and of an intense desire to gratify her needs. She went to her grandparents to satisfy some of these. She modelled her father's loose living and loving. Her great strengths were being submerged by her environment.

Sometimes the children were hit, sometimes they were yelled at; there was no consistency other than the consistency of parents arguing. There were never any one-to-one experiences with mother or father. Her mother only happened to learn of Kelly's inner pain by a surreptitious violation of the privacy of Kelly's diary and was reacting out of fear, not judgement; she felt she was running out of time. One consistent behaviour that survived extinction was mother's dependence on outside professionals. She returned and returned even to the thirteenth try.

It is difficult to describe the process that ensued for the next twelve months, but it began with the insistence of Mr. T's involvement in the process. That was item one in *our* contract. We took a complete inventory of their present situation: their behaviour, Kelly's behaviour, their other daughters' behaviour, their relationship with each other, and their individual relationships with their daughters. On the basis of this inventory, we explored their prediction of what was going to happen to them and to their children. It was a very sad assessment of the present with an equally sad prognosis for the future. This in-depth assessment led to their realization that they were the prime agents of their present state and they had to learn to assume the central role and responsibility for any changes.

They talked, they read, they listened, they cried. The process was slow and often very painful and discouraging. They were learning much about each other and some basic fundamentals of a good contract between themselves. The next stage, after they felt comfortable with their relationship, was an attempt to develop a better understanding and arrangement with their daughters. Where were they to begin to mend and to change years of learning and overlearning of confused values, inconsistent family rules, and negative modelling?

Mrs. and Mrs. T. decided that they would like to share with Kelly their assessment of the present situation and their responsibility for it. They openly communicated their feelings, their regrets, their fears, and their progress in their own relationship and outlined a tentative family plan. It was a plan with well-defined family responsibilities, rules, privileges, freedoms, and procedures to allow for discussion, evaluation, ventilation, and renegotiation. The final contract was to be a product of the total family's input; it would reflect Kelly's needs, her sisters' needs, and the parents' needs and expectations.

They focused on Kelly's strengths and her needs to help develop more appropriate ways of behaviour. Those things that had meaning for her, such as her wish to spend more time taking care of her grandparents and her ambition to become an accomplished guitarist, were used to help her slowly develop her self-discipline and self-esteem. They were growing together.

Mr. and Mrs. T. began to try to develop a one-to-one relationship with Kelly. Mr. T. took Kelly to dinner and a hockey game. He began taping her music and they listened to the tapes together excitedly. Mrs. T. and Kelly decided to take an evening course on design and dressmaking and they began to work together on a new wardrobe for her grandmother.

For the first time the family rented a cottage at the lake for the summer where they had time to look and listen to each other, to work and play together. They all went to church and it began to feel like a religious experience and not a staged performance. As Mrs. T. said, "I feel like a kid with a new toy – my husband and my family. Sometimes I see Kelly sad, distant, and still troubled. She hasn't really let us in yet. I wish ...."

Though there is great resiliency in the young, one cannot erase what sometimes has been indelibly written. The spankings, the threats of abandonment, the punishment, the yelling, the absence of limits, the parental modelling leave scars. Though Mr. and Mrs. T. are much better united and are encouraged by some changes in Kelly, it's too early to know how she will manage her life. In addition to the usual pressures and difficulties of adolescence, Kelly has the weight of a painful history.

Is the case of Kelly and her parents unique or is it a reflection of a more general societal dilemma? Is the high incidence of delinquency, adolescent revolt, generation conflict, disenchantment, and emotional disturbance a consequence of permissive child-rearing, an authoritarian parental regime, or parental ignorance? Whatever the cause, many of life's stresses and failures are a result of lack of self-discipline, self-control, or will power. From whence comes this important self-discipline, this self-control that is so often related to achievement, self-esteem, and stability? Is it an inherited quality or is it learned? If learned, where, how, and in what circumstances?

Definitions of Discipline – New and Old

The old definition of discipline was "to instruct, to educate and to train in mental and moral development; to foster proper conduct and action by instruction and exercise of the instruction." Over time this positive definition has degenerated to its current meaning: "to punish, to control, to subdue, to correct, to thrash, and to chastise." (Oxford)

In a recent survey we asked mothers "does discipline mean: a) to punish, or b) to educate?" Seventy-eight per cent answered that discipline meant "to punish" and 22 per cent answered "to educate." It is unfortunate that discipline has taken on this negative meaning since it is a set of procedures used to teach rules and ways of appropriate and productive behaviour. It is an essential process that takes years with the ultimate goal being the development of socialization skills, social judgement, social roles, *self-discipline*, and *self-control*. If we do not develop our own self-control, we remain fixated at an immature level where we can rely only on external control, external management, policing, and punishment.

Have our present discipline methods in child-rearing resulted in the development of self-discipline in adults? How do we measure it? We have only to look at the incidence of obesity and overweight to find that 30 to 40 per cent of the population are overweight and have not learned self-control even though they are aware of such consequences as diabetes and hypertension. The millions of smokers who don't kick the weed in spite of the established relationship of smoking to cancer and heart attacks also attest to the non-learning of self-discipline, as do the violence, delinquency, alcoholism, drug dependency, child abuse, wife abuse, and many other out-of-control indulgences that have brought grief in family and generational conflicts.

A more than casual reading of the daily newspaper will indicate that (1) we live in a society with millions of adults and adolescents who are fixated at an immature level and who have not developed this self-control; (2) we rely heavily on external policing and punishing controls; and (3) these external controls are not working.

It's difficult for many of us to relate to these problems of self-discipline in our society even though most of us are touched by them. However, as parents we can easily relate to the day-to-day questions of how to manage discipline. What are the do's and don'ts when we are confronted with:

"My three-year-old is always running out on the road."
"He pinches and scratches other kids."
"He just refuses to go to bed."
"She's always reading comic books."

"She doesn't help around the house."

"She has temper tantrums if she doesn't get her way."

"He lies about everything."

These problems are real and frustrating. Parents often look for quick solutions, which very often end up as a whack or some other form of punishment. These may be effective for a short time, but such punishment may have undesirable side effects.

There are guidelines to disciplinary skills that must be learned for the parent to be able to deal with problem behaviour effectively. "Effectively" means that you eventually eliminate the behaviour without any psychological or physical damage to the child and that the child learns an alternative way of behaving that is acceptable and rewarding.

The Right and Wrong Reasons for Discipline

Although there are cultural differences in techniques, the need for discipline is universal. Many authority agents are involved in the disciplinary task, but the earliest and most influential agents are parents. Unfortunately, parents often discipline for the wrong reasons and leave scars because the discipline is more punitive than teaching. The wrong reasons include:

- blowing off steam
- retribution
- dispensing justice in an authoritarian, eye-for-eye manner
- revenge
- establishing authority simply to prove who's boss
- impatience
- displacement of frustration (children are easy targets)
- jealousy

To be sure, there are right reasons as well for discipline. These come under three general categories.

1. *Safety and health.* Discipline is necessary at times to protect a child's safety and health when he is too young to understand the dangers and the consequences of his behaviour.

2. *Socialization.* A child must be taught to conform to family and social norms, to respect the rights of others, and to accept that others have reasonable expectations of him. Discipline can serve a valuable function in assisting this socialization process, i.e., the learning and

126

assumption of roles and responsibilities.

3. *Impulse control and emotional security.* Discipline is necessary for the emotional security of children. Without unambiguous limits and rules to use as standards for impulse control they feel confused and insecure. Without these limits they are under a great strain because of their immaturity and limited degree of self-control. Some children become fearful of their uninhibited behaviour in terms of retribution and guilt. For some, discipline, and specifically punishment, reduces their guilt feelings.

Methods of Discipline

To achieve these goals of discipline, there are four basic methods: reward, punishment, rational explanation, and modelling. It is not a matter of selecting just one of these methods, since the needs of children require that parents have in their repertoire the skill and understanding of *all* these methods of discipline along with the sensitivity as to what method is most appropriate in a given situation. The stage of intellectual, emotional, and social development, the personality of the child, his best style of learning, and the specific situation dictate which combination of methods is preferable.

Basic to these methods is a good family contract which operates as a set of plans for the building of behaviours and relationships. As indicated in Chapter Seven, this contract or agreement must reflect the expectations, needs, motives, and values of *all* members of the family and clearly and explicitly outline rules, roles, and responsibilities, and the consequences of misbehaviour. The contract must be fair, flexible, sensitive to age and stage, must have specific procedures for when, where, and how a family member ventilates his suggestions or complaints or renegotiates the terms of the contract.

Since there are individual differences and peculiarities in perception and memory of what decisions were made, it is suggested that much of the contract be written out to avoid, "I didn't think that *I* was responsible for cutting the lawn all summer, digging the flower beds, taking out the garbage, and feeding the dog – I thought Abe Lincoln freed the slaves."

RATIONAL EXPLANATION

The role of rational explanation in the development of discipline is to instruct and teach: to clearly state what the expected behaviour is, why it's required, and the consequences of misbehaviour. It also includes the exploration and suggestions of behaviours alternative to undesirable behaviour. For example, if you are talking on the phone and your child keeps interrupting, crying, and trying obnoxiously to get your attention, you have a number of alternatives:

1. *Hit or yell at him to "shut up and keep quiet."* Neither one of you feels very good after this method and it generally results in short-term effectiveness and long-term side effects (discussed under punishment).
2. *Ignore the interruptions and the noise* – it may cease or increase the intensity of the interruptions. This method will be discussed further in Chapter Eleven.
3. *Try to divert his attention.* "Go have a cookie or watch television" usually works for a short period only.
4. *Ask the person to whom you are talking to hold on for a moment.* Don't terminate the call and say you will call back, since terminating the call is exactly what your child would like and this reinforces the irritating behaviour. Explain to your child: "This is an important call. I want to talk to this person without interruption. Interruption makes me angry. When I finish my telephone call I will listen to whatever you have to say and what you want. I really appreciate your waiting until I'm through. Thank you." This is delivered in a warm, even-toned manner.

The difference between the "shut up" and the rational message has been studied by a number of researchers in child development and they have found that children who grow up in a home where there is rational explanation have more self-discipline, better self-esteem, and their language development is more advanced than it is in children from the one-liner, "shut-up" environments. They also tend to model this approach in their interaction with their siblings and friends.

MODELLING AND IMITATION

If a "do as I say, not as I do" message characterizes the parents' teaching it also necessitates a heavy parental power method of discipline. Eventually the child becomes disappointed in his parents, angry, confused, and insecure about "what really is the proper behaviour." This dissonant message does not teach self-discipline or the correct behaviour; it teaches a child that if you have the power or authority you can get away with anything. "Dad hits me every time he catches me lying, yet he and Mom admit that they lie in special situations. They sure have a lot of special situations."

It is well-established that one of the most powerful modes of learning for children is by imitation and the most influential models in their developing years are the parents. They mimic everything – they put on your clothes, talk like you, walk like you, pretend they really are Mommy or Daddy. By imitation they are (1) saying that they would like to be like you, and (2) trying out and experimenting with new ways of behaving.

Since you are the "Great Model" and the "Great Example," check your behaviour and your own self-discipline. There are some copycats out there learning and duplicating your behaviour. They are also sometimes sickened and antagonized by the inconsistencies in your behaviour and your expectations. They have sensitive radar equipment and it begins to operate very early in their development.

Having indicated that modelling is so important in the teaching and learning of self-discipline we must remember the Learning-Hope Curve (Chapter 3) and that we can't expect instant learning from instant modelling of good behaviour. Learning follows a lawful course and it takes time, faith, encouragement, and a good example.

REWARDS

Though this method will be dealt with extensively in Chapter 9, on behaviour management, it also does teach discipline. If we use the historic definition of discipline, to teach, then we must encourage and strengthen appropriate behaviours. We do this by reinforcement or rewards, such as praise, affection, recognition, or privilege.

As parents we too often focus and overstress negative behaviours while taking for granted or failing to acknowledge the desirable behaviours. A basic human need is the acknowledgement of our appropriate behaviour. It is essential for learning, for emotional security, and for the growth of our self-esteem. In the case of Kelly, it took prodding to get Mrs. T. to acknowledge her strengths. This is a dangerous counter-productive attitude. One begins to change behaviour when one concentrates on a child's strengths. Stop, look, listen, and take the time to reinforce the good things your children do. It becomes a habit and a style and can have important implications. There is often an infectiousness to this style, i.e., when you begin to see and appreciate the good things your children do, they do more good things because your recognition gives them good feelings about themselves. When you start the day like a prison guard checking out the bad actors and looking for bad actions – if you haven't already found them, this attitude will create them.

PUNISHMENT

Is it good? Is it bad? Is it necessary? When do you punish? What type of punishment? What are your alternatives to punishment?

It's good and necessary if (1) it is effective in *completely* extinguishing an inappropriate behaviour; (2) if there is consonant learning of an appropriate behaviour; and (3) if there are no damaging side effects. Although types of punishment are necessary and effective in specific situations, there is overwhelming evidence of the ineffectiveness of harsh punishment and of its disastrous consequences. Parents should be aware of both possibilities and explore their options, and they must be sensitive to the emotional and physical condition of the child. Some children, for example, may have to be spanked occasionally; for others, within the same family, a similar spanking could cause untold damage. Types of punishment include the following:

- physical punishment – spanking, slapping, shaking, etc.
- verbal punishment – yelling, nagging, embarrassing, insulting, belittling
- withdrawal of love and affection
- ignoring behaviour or inattention to the child
- taking away privileges, e.g., toys, trips, TV time
- banishment to room

Before exploring the effectiveness or ineffectiveness and the consequences of these methods of punishment, it's important to recognize the parents' needs and motives to punish. As has been indicated, there are right reasons and wrong reasons for disciplining and the wrong ones are most often followed by physical punishment, e.g., for revenge, to blow off steam, to dispense harsh justice and establish and demonstrate who is boss. These reasons generally do not result in change of behaviour, as is evidenced clearly by the history of our penal system. Punishment may for a short time postpone behaviours but rarely changes or eliminates them.

What Types of Punishment Work? When? and How?

SPANKING

Spanking may have to be used for safety or health reasons, e.g., when a young child runs out on a busy street, plays with electrical outlets, jumps around in a moving boat, lights matches, or pounds a sibling. Spanking or hand-slapping in these situations is often necessary for a very young child (one to four years of age), whose reasoning ability is not as yet developed. He makes an association between the sting of the spanking and the running out on the road. He may not understand that it is dangerous, but he does learn that if he does it, it is followed immediately by discomfort. It is important for the parent, in addition to the spanking, also to begin to explain, even at this early stage of little understanding, the reasons why this behaviour is dangerous. It demonstrates respect for the child and though the child may not understand, the tone and firmness of voice begin to make an impression. It also establishes a pattern for future parental treatment and intervention in problem behaviour. It establishes a good *habit*. The meaning of "no" is also established if "no" is used at the same instant as the running out on the road and the spanking. The "no," by association, takes on the power of the spanking and becomes a cue or a deterrent.

Note: a physical beating which injures the child is abuse, not punishment. A spanking is not the same thing as a beating. A parent who causes anything more serious than brief pinkness and a stinging sensation has committed a serious offence against his or her child. A parent who repeats such an offence should seek professional help *immediately*.

VERBAL PUNISHMENT

Yelling, nagging, embarrassing, insulting, and belittling may stop a behaviour for a very short time, but such verbal punishment very rarely eliminates the bad behaviour. When yelling stops an undesirable behaviour it reinforces the parent and yelling becomes a habit! However, there are circumstances in which you have the right to be angry and to raise your voice.

The sequence: Carole has a temper tantrum. You yell. She stops. One of the reasons may be that you are finally paying attention to her. For her the temper tantrum worked and so she has learned that to get your attention all she has to do is have a tantrum. You feel good because the tantrum stopped and you have learned that to stop such behaviour all you have to do is yell at her. One hour later she has another temper tantrum and you yell and yell and become Old Yeller.

The consequence: You have not eliminated the behaviour (temper tantrums) but have developed an equally obnoxious, ineffective behaviour. Another danger is that this behaviour may be modelled. You have the responsibility of exploring the reasons for the temper tantrums and of seeking a more constructive method of dealing with them.

As a reaction to an inappropriate behaviour, parents sometimes resort to insult or belittlement. The result of this attack is usually the development of poor self-esteem.

Deal with the "bad behaviour" but don't label the child "bad." "I love you, but I don't like what you are doing now." Avoid saying, "You are a bad boy (or girl)." Such a label can damage self-esteem, and there is a self-fulfilling prophecy to labels.

WITHDRAWAL OF LOVE AND AFFECTION

Parental love, affection, and warmth should not be negotiable. One can be upset, angry, and take away privileges but should not treat love as a privilege. The withdrawal of love as a punishment will cause emotional insecurity, problems with close interpersonal relationships, and neurotic behaviour.

WITHDRAWAL OF PRIVILEGES

Privileges for appropriate behaviour and consequences of misbehaviour should be fair, clear, explicit, and well-communicated in a parent-child contract. Don't make up all the rules as you go along. Withdrawal of privileges can be very effective if administered immediately following inappropriate behaviour or a breach in your parent-child contract. Along with the withdrawal of privileges it is important that a rational explanation and discussion take place with an exploration into alternative behaviours.

SOME DANGERS OF PHYSICAL PUNISHMENT

Although, as noted earlier, physical punishment at times may be necessary, there are a number of dangers in this form of punishment besides the obvious danger of an out-of-control parent becoming a child abuser. These dangers include the following.

1. Fear and anxiety are by-products of physical punishment especially. This fear can be generalized to other people and other situations and may last a lifetime. Children tend to resist physical punishment by learning to fight back.
2. Such punishment can destroy present and future parent-child relationships. Children begin to avoid a punishing parent.
3. It acts as a model, i.e., children learn to hit and use physical punishment and become aggressive.
4. It can create passivity, overconformity, and withdrawal.
5. Fears of punishment may stifle creativity, enthusiasm, openness, and co-operation.
6. It damages self-esteem.
7. Children learn to escape punishment by avoiding places associated with physical punishment, e.g., the home or school.
8. Neurotic or maladjusted behaviour is learned when a child receives frequent punishment and can't escape it.

9. Punishment may become reinforcing if a child accepts it as a form of attention. Consequently, the undesirable behaviour increases.
10. It quickly reduces guilt and can become reinforcing because of the quick absolution. This may retard a child's moral development.
11. Physical punishment does not teach new and more appropriate behaviours.
12. Parents often punish because they don't know a better way to deal with the behaviour, or because they cannot control their anger and hostility.

Suggestions and Rules for Discipline

The discipline of children inevitably involves the question of "What shall I do in this spontaneous and immediate situation?" With the following suggestions and rules firmly in mind, the parent will not be able to change the immediacy and spontaneity of behaviours that require discipline; these suggestions and rules, however, should help to free the parent from his or her own spontaneously irrational response to the misbehaviour. Above all, remember that the purpose of discipline should be to teach.

1. Develop a contract with your child so that you are not operating from crisis to crisis.
2. Be consistent. If a behaviour is treated as acceptable one day but not the next, the behaviour will not disappear. Also, if you warn a child not to do something or there will be a consequence and he proceeds to do it anyway, don't then decide that you can't be bothered. Follow through with the consequence or you will be *more bothered* later. And don't make vague threats and warnings you are not prepared to follow through if necessary. The frequent lapse into the "or else" syndrome can be self-defeating. Your inconsistency will cause conflict and antisocial behaviour in your child.
3. You can criticize an act or behaviour, but don't follow with insult or an attack on the child's personality and self-concept. You can call it a bad act, but you don't have to attach the label "you're a bad kid" to it.
4. Deal with the present situation, don't dig up history.
5. Your discipline should be appropriate to the child's level of age, stage, and understanding.
6. You can't always be popular. If the contract requires a consequence, don't back down for fear of loss of your child's love.

7. Instruction is more effective than punishment.
8. Model the behaviour you would like to see in your children.
9. Differentiate between intentional acts and accidental acts.
10. Using peer discipline and peer pressure often results in less resistance.
11. Hesitation in enforcing a consequence of a misdemeanour can cause frustration in you and conflict in the child. If you have adequately assessed the behaviour as inappropriate, deal with it! Uncertainty about what you will do creates anxiety additional to the guilt and anxiety he likely has because of the misbehaviour.
12. Is your perception of the behaviour accurate? A number of factors affect your perception, such as your present physical or emotional condition and other stressors. If you have just had an argument with your wife and your daughter comes in and slams the door (perhaps accidentally), your perception of that act can be affected by your emotional state.
13. To differentiate acceptable and non-acceptable behaviour, parents have found it helpful to use Dr. Fritz Redl's notion of red light, green light, and yellow light behaviours. Green light behaviours are acceptable; red light behaviours are unacceptable; yellow light behaviours are acceptable only under special conditions. Children can identify with this. Make a list of red, green, and yellow behaviours with your child. It is not only a contract they can understand, but they will enjoy being part of the development of the contract.
14. Remember the Learning-Hope Curve. It takes time to learn a new behaviour and even though you may not see immediate outward performance, learning is going on inside the child.
15. Your *prime* goal in discipline is to ensure that your child will move from the elementary, primitive stage of the external control of his behaviour to the mature stage of *self-discipline* and *self-control* of his behaviour.

Styles of Parental Discipline

Perhaps one of the most instructive research studies was carried out by Diana Baumrind, who identified three different child-rearing styles and their effects. *Authoritative parents* were firm but warm, non-rejecting, willing to explain and reconsider rules. Their children turned out to be the most competent, self-reliant, self-controlled, and content. *Authoritarian parents* were detached, power-oriented, highly controlling, restrictive, over-protective, and unwilling to discuss or reconsider rules. Their children were less competent, discontented, withdrawn, and distrustful. *Permissive parents* were non-controlling and non-demanding, with no firm rules established. Their children turned out to be the least competent, dependent, aimless, and irresponsible.

Baumrind's research indicates that the attributes of competence, independence, outgoingness, self-control, and self-reliance are fostered by supportive, warm home environments in which independent actions and decision-making as well as responsible and self-reliant behaviour are modelled, encouraged, and rewarded. Parents who combine high but reasonable maturity demands, clearly defined standards of behaviour with open communication and explanations of the reason for these standards (but who do not use arbitrary authoritarian discipline, severe punitiveness, and overprotection) promote the development of maturity, competence, and socially responsible children.

Finally, discipline should not be equated with punishment. Discipline is a parent's positive attitude to child behaviours that have to be *learned* in two stages. The learning of discipline begins with teaching and guidance and the monitoring of one's behaviour by outside agents – primarily parents – and matures to a stage of self-control and self-discipline. Millions of adults are fixated at the immature stage, where performance, conformity, and control have to be policed by external agents. The consequence of this fixation is a lack of self-discipline which is reflected by the high incidence of overweight, smoking, alcohol and drug abuse, divorce, criminal acts, and academic and job failures. The kind of discipline you use as a parent will be a significant factor in the kind of adult (and parent) your child becomes.

NINE

Behaviour Management:
The Art and Science of Motivation

It is difficult to explain a simple behavioral approach which rests on direct, immediate consequences and not on intriguing deceptions.

It is difficult to understand that the question of discipline is not one of strictness or permissiveness but one of cause and effect relationships.
— **CLIFFORD K. MADSEN and CHARLES H. MADSEN, JR.**

The therapeutic methods derived from these principles cannot be learned overnight or merely by reading a do "it" yourself manual. Effective behavior modification requires sensitivity to the most subtle cues.
— **REDD, PORTERFIELD, and ANDERSON**

A System for Answering the Persistent Questions of Parents

How do I motivate my child to:

- do homework
- read a book
- go to bed on time
- clean her/his room
- wash and brush
- set the table
- pick up toys
- take better care of possessions
- help around the house
- share ....

How do I deal with:

- hitting
- teasing
- lying
- swearing
- whining
- interrupting
- temper tantrums
- selfishness
- destructiveness
- constant TV watching
- aggression
- fearfulness ....

BEHAVIOUR MANAGEMENT

Behaviour management is a powerful system of teaching that includes certain tried-and-proven principles for motivating people, together with a set of procedures for putting these principles into practice. Using these principles and procedures, you can teach your children behaviours that you consider appropriate and that reflect your values. You can, in the process, help your children to become more independent, creative, and productive while eliminating their undesirable behaviour.

Behaviour management is derived from learning theory and is based on thousands of experiments and research studies that have confirmed the system's validity. The system is practical and can be dramatically effective. However, time must be invested to learn its methods. The learning process also requires a commitment by both parents to become actively involved, to agree on the procedures, and to be consistent in their administration. Behaviour management does not suggest or propose *what* behaviours you should change or develop. Such decisions are yours, to be based on your own personal values as well as those of your child. One concern sometimes voiced even by proponents of behaviour management is that, if a parent's motives are selfish or pathological or otherwise open to question, there is danger that behaviours may be encouraged which are not in the child's best interests. Our assumption throughout this discussion is that parents are motivated positively and always with the child's best interests and needs uppermost in mind. There are six basic principles of behaviour management.

1. Most behaviour is learned.

2. Learned behaviours can be unlearned.

3. Reinforcement increases the probability of a behaviour.

4. Intermittent reward strengthens behaviour.

5. Reward each small step toward a goal.

6. Negative reinforcement helps to terminate undesirable behaviour.

Principle 1: Most Behaviour is Learned

Almost all behaviours are *learned* – the good as well as the bad. Picking up toys, sharing, enjoying reading, completing homework, and helping around the house are examples of the good behaviours that can be learned. Temper tantrums, lying, swearing, fear of water, being late for school, and overeating are examples of bad behaviours that can be learned. Some behaviours, generally called "reflexive," are not learned. In this category are such behaviours as an eye blink, a knee jerk, and other reflexes and behaviours that may be traced to injuries or illnesses, including metabolic, glandular, and central nervous system disorders.

Principle 2: Behaviours Can Be Unlearned

Behaviour management also states that it is possible to *unlearn* a learned behaviour. This basic principle applies to both the good and bad behaviours. The following principles demonstrate how behaviour can be strengthened or weakened.

Principle 3: Positive Reinforcement

Any behaviour followed *immediately* by a positive reinforcer is "streng-thened." That is, such behaviour is more likely to occur again than a behaviour which has not been strengthened. A positive reinforcer is, in essence, a reward. Though we commonly think of such material things as money, prizes, trips, stars, toys, candy, and other tangible objects as rewards there are other rewards – called *social reinforcers* – that can be even more powerful in motivating children. Among these are parental attention, expressions of love, recognition, approval, a smile, a pat, or a hug.

A reward, to be truly rewarding, must be something *you* personally desire, something that will cause *you* to act, an object or an action that is meaningful to *you*. What is a reward for Mary may not necessarily be a reward for John, or vice versa. Mary might consider a trip to McDonald's a reward, but for John (who hates hamburgers) such a trip would be a punishment. Sue enjoys doing the grocery shopping for her mother because she enjoys her mother's reaction afterwards – the thanks, the hugs, the smile. Claire, on the other hand, shops for her mother because she is paid $1.50 for every shopping trip, and Claire is saving up for a visit to New York.

Sue's motives are considered "intrinsic"; Claire's motives are termed "extrinsic." You may prefer to encourage either type, or both types, of action. What is important to note at this point is that – in the examples cited – *both* intrinsic and extrinsic motivations achieved the desired goal: to get the grocery shopping accomplished.

Which motive is better? We like to believe that all behaviour should be intrinsic and that people should do things for the sheer joy or goodness of the act itself. Unfortunately, life doesn't work that way, and to assume that it does is to ignore the facts and the laws of nature. To cite an example, Peter likes his job because it's interesting and challenging, and he knows that good performance is always rewarded by positive feedback from the boss. These are his *intrinsic* rewards. But Peter also is paid $35,000 a year, works in a beautiful office, and enjoys many fringe benefits. These are his *extrinsic* rewards. If his company stopped giving Peter his *extrinsic* rewards (his pay, office, and benefits), Peter would quit – even if the boss doubled up on the *intrinsic* rewards (the compliments and back pats). Real life involves a combination of extrinsic and intrinsic rewards and motives. Hence, parents who expect their children to act strictly for altruistic reasons, and to react solely to non-tangible rewards, are being neither fair nor realistic.

Dad and Mom work hard for both extrinsic and intrinsic compensations. Why, then, should they apply different criteria to their children, who also may work hard in discharging their chores and responsibilities? In terms of reinforcement, is there any real difference between Dad's or Mom's bonus at work and their daughter's $1.50 reward for doing the shopping? Toys, money, attention, praise, trips, and affection are all reinforcers. They all work, and they all motivate children as much as they motivate grown-ups.

When choosing a reinforcer, consult your child. Your perception of what is reinforcing may differ from your child's perception. If your concept is faulty, any reinforcer based upon it cannot promote or strengthen the desired behaviour. Remember, also, that you cannot legislate what reward should be meaningful to your child, or to anyone else, merely by the force of your will. Motivations and rewards have deeply personal meanings that vary from person to person. You will need to be continually and acutely alert, listening to and observing your children's words and actions with great care, if you hope to bring about important, long-lasting changes.

The principle of positive reinforcement is not new; it has been used – consciously or unconsciously – by parents and teachers for a long time. Unfortunately, the principle often is applied inconsistently or incorrectly. An example of inconsistency may be found in many class-rooms. Teachers may, for example, award stars, marks, and privileges as incentives for learning and performance. The same teachers also may recognize the power of social reinforcers, using attention, approval, verbal praise, and affection as rewards. However, according to Harvard University studies, some teachers spend too much time positively reinforcing the high achievers and too little time boosting the slow learners, even when the latter have performed adequately. Slow learners, according to the Harvard researchers, are much more likely to receive negative or zero reinforcement than are the high achievers. The same imbalance often is found in the home as well as in the classroom. Why? Because high achievers, in turn, reinforce parents and teachers. They fulfil our needs and reinforce our motives. The behaviour of high achievers demonstrates that we are competent, successful teachers (or parents). Children who are slow to learn, and who cannot read, are an embarrassment; they demonstrate that we have failed as teachers (or parents). We thus feel threatened – a negative reinforcement. When a child performs well in the presence of a visiting principal, the teacher takes the credit; he or she is perceived as the agent responsible for the student's good performance, and the teacher wins a reward (commendation) from his or her supervisor.

In sum, the children who need reinforcement the most get it the least!

CAN WE LEARN TO BE BETTER REINFORCERS?

Some people are, by instinct or training, better reinforcers than others. They are more sensitive to the needs of others and have developed the ability to pay careful attention to others, to listen intently, to look directly at others, to praise, and to empathize. People like to be with individuals who have these abilities.

Can we learn to become better social reinforcers? Fortunately, the answer appears to be "yes." One interesting study conducted in a midwestern school system demonstrated dramatically that teachers can become more effective as social reinforcers. In the school system under study, teachers were informed that the extent to which they used such reinforcers in Week One would be measured by the researchers. During the same week, the investigators also measured class productivity in terms of correct answers on assignments. In Week Two, the teachers were asked to step up their use of social reinforcers – praise, smiles, attention, and the like – by approximately 25 per cent. Class productivity was again measured in Week Two and was found to have increased significantly. After a month of these experiments, the teachers were asked to return to their Week One level of reinforcement. When they decreased the smiles, pats, hugs, and other reinforcers to the original level, productivity (as measured by the number of correct answers) fell *below* the level of Week One. These results, obtained under controlled conditions, forcibly demonstrated the effectiveness of social reinforcers as incentives to learning and performance.

ARE REWARDS BRIBERY?

Some parents and teachers say they are uncomfortable with the concept of rewards. They argue that rewards are really a form of bribery. The answer to this criticism is that most parents and teachers already are using reinforcers and rewards every day, at home and in school, but are using them inappropriately rather than according to the scientific principles of learning theory and behaviour management.

Webster's New International Dictionary defines bribery, in part, as "the act of influencing the action of another by corrupt inducement." The same source defines "bribe" as a "price, reward, gift, or favor bestowed or promised with a view to pervert the judgment or corrupt the conduct of a person in a position of trust." It certainly is not the intent of reinforcement when used by teachers or parents to pervert or corrupt conduct. The objective of positive reinforcement, correctly used, is to increase or strengthen appropriate behaviour.

DON'T TAKE GOOD BEHAVIOUR FOR GRANTED

When you use this principle of positive reinforcement for behaviour, you are saying, in substance, "That was good behaviour. I want it to happen again. Therefore, I will reward this behaviour immediately, to strengthen it." If your child picks up his or her toys and puts them in the appropriate storage area, *don't take this act for granted*. This is a behaviour you want to be repeated. Praise the child for it; give him or her a hug. The child enjoys and welcomes such recognition and the hug. Also, the child learns how to get *you* to behave and react. In other words, the child is reinforcing – in *you* – the praising and hugging behaviour, and strengthening it.

The process is not, of course, limited to children. When my wife thanks me for clearing the table or helping with the dishes her thanks make me feel good. Even though I accept that such acts are part of my responsibility around the house, I like her affectionate reaction.

Do not assume that a single reinforcement will establish a desired behaviour. Usually, many reinforcements are required over a period of time. It is vitally important, also, to remember that your children look to you as a model. If you, as a parent, pick up your "toys," this serves to strengthen further the child's learning of that behaviour. It is axiomatic that one of the best ways to learn is by imitation. Young children want to dress like you, talk like you, act like you, *be* like you.

LOVE AS A REINFORCER

Note that when the use of social reinforcers is suggested (attention, praise, a hug, and the like), we do not use the word "love" among such reinforcers. There may, indeed, be love involved in praise, a hug, smile, or other reinforcers. But in the earlier chapter on discipline it was stressed that *love is not negotiable.* "Mommy will love you if you eat your cereal, and Mommy will not love you if you don't." Such an abuse of the concept of love forces the child to place little value on a feeling that is negotiable in such small transactions. The end result can be emotional insecurity in the child, who may then regard any behaviour involving love with suspicion.

USING REINFORCERS AS "STARTERS"

Sometimes when a child has difficulty with learning a certain skill, he will avoid behaviour associated with that learning. For example, a child who is failing in reading may simply stop trying to read. The resultant failure leaves him hurt and frustrated, and his self-confidence suffers a crippling blow. In such instances, a reinforcer may be used as a "starter" to reactivate the child's interest in learning. If the reinforcer is personally meaningful to him – perhaps it is a much desired toy, or a trip to some favoured spot – he will make an initial effort to read again. This is Stage 1 in a three-stage process. At the same time you are encouraging him with a tangible reward, you can also reinforce him "socially" with praise or attention. This is Stage 2. Note carefully that you are "pairing" or associating the toy or the trip with the social reinforcer (a pat, hug, or other sign of approval). Finally, when the child begins to succeed in his efforts to read, he begins also to enjoy the act of reading, and reading in itself becomes intrinsically rewarding. This is Stage 3 – the payoff.

Principle 4: Intermittent Reward Strengthening Behaviour

CONTINUOUS REINFORCEMENT

To establish a behaviour, the learner should be reinforced every time he

142

performs or shows improvement. You reinforce *every time* and *immediately* after the behaviour. But do you need to reinforce every time forever? There is a potential problem at this point: if behaviour is learned under this continuous-reward schedule, the behaviour ultimately will cease if you discontinue the rewards. To avoid this eventuality, once the behaviour is established you can switch to intermittent reinforcement.

INTERMITTENT REINFORCEMENT

This regimen encourages a child to continue an established behaviour despite a gradual decrease in the frequency with which the behaviour is reinforced. Instead of rewarding every performance, you begin to reinforce the behaviour every other time it occurs. You then consciously switch the reinforcing schedule to one of intermittent intervals, rewarding the child at (say) every third or sixth occurrence, then back to every fourth, and so on. By design, you stretch out the intervals between rewards.

For example, assume that the desired behaviour is putting away toys. At the outset, you reward the child every time he puts his toys away. You find that the behaviour becomes established after the child performs and is rewarded six nights in a row. You then move into an intermittent schedule in which – for one week – you reinforce the learner every other night after he puts his toys away. During the second week, you reward him on, say, Monday, Wednesday, Thursday, and Sunday, that is, on an irregular basis with progressively longer intervals between rewards. This is a powerful method of establishing and maintaining behaviour.

In sum, reinforcement should be as continuous as possible at the beginning. But in the real world, rewarding the learner every time is obviously not possible, so you reinforce as close to this ideal schedule as you can. Continuous reinforcement results in rapid learning, but intermittent reinforcement makes behaviours strong, persistent, and resistant to extinction. Behaviours reinforced randomly, say, every fourth time, will persist longer than behaviours that have been reinforced continuously.

USING TOKENS AND POINTS AS REINFORCERS

Some reinforcers are readily available and portable, including such social rewards as a smile, a hug, and other forms of attention. These, and such tangible rewards as money and candy, can be delivered immediately following a desired behaviour. But many rewards are not available for immediate delivery and must be promised for future payment. If a child must wait two hours, a day, or a month for the promised reinforcer, it loses its strength. For this reason, you can introduce a *token* reinforcer, which can be delivered immediately.

Tokens that have been used successfully with children include stars, poker chips, check marks, and points. These can be converted into real rewards, such as a book, a toy, a trip, or some special privilege. Our entire economic system operates on tokens. Our pay cheques, pieces of paper with no intrinsic value whatsoever, are tokens to be traded for material objects or services. In like fashion, reinforcer tokens have no value in themselves but may be traded for rewards. For example, a child may earn five tokens, permitting him to watch TV for thirty minutes; earn five tokens, for which a parent will read him a story; earn ten tokens, which "buy"a trip to Dad's office where the child may use the typewriter; earn ten tokens, for a kite; earn twenty tokens, for a hockey game; earn fifty tokens, for a camping trip.

The obvious advantage of this token system is that it allows you to reward the child immediately after the desired behaviour. Tokens also teach the learner to delay his need gratification, that is, to work for a certain period before he is rewarded with something he considers important and valuable. Most achievers and successful people have learned to wait, to work for their need and to delay their gratification. Conversely, many dropouts and delinquents seek immediate gratification of their needs – they must have the payoff *right now*.

Our society understands the token principle and relies upon it every day to elicit desired behaviour. Millions of adults save trading stamps, which they ultimately exchange for tangible rewards (reinforcers), and grocery discount coupons, which they exchange for cash savings at the supermarket. Most children at one time or another collect tokens – baseball or football cards, for example – which may be traded for books, toys, dolls, or other objects. In applying the token system to a behaviour problem, then, you are merely applying a principle that has already proven its effectiveness in our everyday life.

BEHAVIOUR CONTRACTS

To eliminate reliance on memory, a written contract should be prepared. The contract should be clear and explicit (see Chapter 8 for details). Parents should discuss and agree upon its provisions with respect to the specific behaviour desired and the specific rewards to be granted. If a token arrangement is involved, a provision can also be included under which the child *loses* tokens for inappropriate behaviour. The contract, agreed to and perhaps signed by all parties concerned, should be valid for a specified period of time, at the end of which the agreement may be evaluated and renegotiated.

Principle 5: Reward Each Small Step toward a Goal

This principle suggests that parents assess each desired behaviour to determine whether the child is capable, physically or intellectually, of learning and performing it. The behaviour may be too complex and beyond a child's ability. You must begin where the child's skills are. Set up a program by breaking the behaviour into small steps. The child is then reinforced for every small step toward the final desired behaviour. Your child's performance will guide you as to how big or small the steps should be.

Mother, for example, would like eight-year-old Trudy to make her own bed. She leaves it in a big mess every morning. In taking inventory of the situation, Mother recognizes that the bedspread is too heavy for her, and it is also beyond her physical ability to lift the mattress and tuck the sheets in. The first step was to have Trudy just pull up her blanket over the bed. It didn't matter how straight it was. This was easy for Trudy and she was immediately reinforced for this first success by a hug and an extra half hour of TV that day. The next step included pulling up the blanket over her bed and straightening her pillows. The third step was to smooth out her sheets, cover her bed with her blanket, and straighten the pillows. Her mother helped her by demonstration. Mother replaced the heavy bedspread with a very light manageable one and Trudy was ready for the final step, the bedspread. Every step was within her capability and she was reinforced as she succeeded. It was a great triumph for Trudy and her entire family shared the excitement of her accomplishment.

Or consider George. According to George's school report he is not doing his homework assignments and is failing. His teacher suggests that George must do at least one and a half hours of homework each evening to get caught up with the rest of the class. Since at the moment he isn't doing any homework, the expectation of one and a half hours is unrealistic. He has not learned to sit and study in his room at all. It will take small successive steps to reach the desired goal. A contract is developed between George and his parents and Step One in the contract is ten minutes of homework per night for the first week. The reinforcement may include praise and tokens toward a new bike. Step Two may be fifteen minutes of homework. Step Three may be thirty minutes. If thirty minutes is too long, they go back to twenty minutes. The time is increased according to his development of homework skills, not his parents' impatient expectations. The reinforcement, which at first was for just attempting to sit and to do his homework, eventually may take into account some measure of productivity, e.g., grades on his next report card.

If a contract is not working, it could be because the steps are beyond the child's capacity or the reinforcers are not meaningful. Evaluate the contract and renegotiate the steps and the reinforcement. When the child begins to achieve, this feeling of success will take over as the reinforcement.

Principle 6: Negative Reinforcement

To weaken an undesirable behaviour it must be followed immediately by an adverse outcome, which is seen by the child as a punishment and which the child can terminate by a change in his or her behaviour.

ELIMINATING UNDESIRABLE BEHAVIOUR

So far we have concentrated on the learning and strengthening of desirable behaviours. As parents, we know well that many child behaviours are inappropriate or obnoxious and give us concern. Before considering the alternatives available for eliminating an inappropriate behaviour, subject that behaviour to an "ABC analysis." A represents the Antecedent, or cause, of the behaviour. B represents the inappropriate Behaviour. C stands for the Consequence of this behaviour. For example,

A. During the family dinner, you are listening to and talking with Paul, while Dad chats with Mary. No one pays any attention to little Joe.

B. Joe plays with his food, then turns his plate upside down.

C. Dad yells at Joe, or slaps his bottom, or both.

If the Consequence – the yell and / or the slap – eliminates the behaviour, you have solved the problem. Chances are, however, that such will not be the case. Even if Joe does not flip his food over the next time he makes a bid for attention, he may try some other inappropriate or obnoxious act. In this case, C did not work because (1) it was not an effective, long-lasting solution, and (2) it did not consider A, which was the cause of B. What motivated Joe to dump his plate? Had Joe's behaviour been subjected to an immediate ABC analysis, you might have decided to pay more attention to Joe and to include him in the family discussions. In other words, you might have eliminated B by changing A.

Trying to understand A is the logical beginning. If a change in A does not eliminate the undesirable behaviour, assess the effectiveness of C (in this instance, the yell and / or the slap). Did it work? For how long? Did C create other problems later? If C didn't work, and Joe continues to pull the dials off the TV set (or whatever), what other C's are available?

It will be to your advantage to take the time to perform these simple analyses, as they can become highly useful problem-solving tools. Our survey of over 600 parents disclosed that 70 per cent of those questioned used physical punishment, even though they did not feel it was effective in the long run. "It's a way of letting my anger out," said one parent.

But there are better ways! Here are six alternatives.

SIX ALTERNATIVE METHODS

Behaviour management includes at least six formal methods for decreasing or eliminating undesirable behaviours. These can be used individually and sometimes may be employed effectively in combination. They are:

- satiation
- ignoring
- non-reward
- punishment
- negative reinforcement
- rewarding alternative desirable behaviours

Each of these methods is based on substantial evidence of success derived from psychological experimentation.

"Undesirable behaviour" can be a relative term, of course. What may be undesirable to the Johnsons may *not* appear undesirable to the Jacksons. A behaviour that may be seen as very serious to one teacher may not be viewed as a problem by another. Standards, values, experience, skills, and your stress level often determine what behaviour is undesirable and under what circumstances. The following are some of the undesirable behaviours for which parents frequently ask help: temper tantrums, bed-wetting, thumb-sucking, whining, defiance, lying, swearing, stealing, fighting, fear of the dark, fear of water, smoking, overeating, playing with matches, and sloppiness.

THE SATIATION METHOD

Allow the child to continue acting out the undesirable behaviour. This may prove effective because (a) the child gets no negative reaction from you, that is, the child is trying to "get your goat" and is failing; (b) the child grows bored with his own behaviour; or (c) the child becomes exhausted or fatigued by his own behaviour. The satiation method may be used when the behaviour does not pose any danger to the child or to others. It is often effective for such behaviours as rude language, incessant talking, eating junk foods, or refusal to go to bed on time.

For example, "Peter, you seem to really enjoy using the word 's---.' Why don't you sit down here, and just use it for as long as you want. Don't stop. I want you to repeat it for at least two hours." Exhaustion, boredom, or the mere failure to get a parent's "goat" may well bring about the end of the undesirable behaviour. In this situation, you would also attempt to reinforce alternative *desirable* behaviours while trying to put an end to the *undesirable*. You would reinforce Peter for verbal behaviour (cleaned-up language) as appropriate.

Parents often look for and "catch" bad behaviour. Try also to "catch" and reward good behaviour. Don't take good behaviour for granted. This child is a developing organism. You are the shaper and teacher, not a policeman.

THE IGNORING METHOD

Many child psychologists maintain that the prime reason for a young child's inappropriate behaviour is the youngster's *need for attention*. When a child interrupts, whines, or throws a temper tantrum, and your response is a reinforcement (a hug or smile or, as the case may be, a yell or a slap), the child's undesirable behaviour has paid off – you are now paying attention. In this case, the child is succcessfully reinforcing and shaping the parent's behaviour.

A typical scenario may go something like this:

1. you are talking on the phone;
2. your child wants attention;
3. she whines;
4. you terminate or interrupt your phone call, perhaps abruptly;
5. you shout at her; and
6. she stops whining.

Your yelling has been reinforced because it stopped the whining. But the whining has also been strengthened – "all I have to do to get her attention and to hang up the phone is to whine." Your child has not learned how to gain your attention in a more positive manner. Ignoring an undesirable behaviour is a more productive option. A child learns he cannot get your attention by whining.

At times you may find it very difficult to wait for the behaviour to stop. Keep your cool. Leave the room, if necessary. Try not to show any concern or emotion. A child learns, after five, six, or maybe ten repetitions, that whining or temper tantrums do not work. It is your responsibility to encourage and reinforce positive behaviours, and to fulfil his need for attention.

Ignoring can be a valuable and powerful technique for eliminating negative behaviour. If physical harm or damage to persons or property results from such behaviour, you obviously would not ignore that kind of behaviour. You would need, in this instance, to resort to one of the other methods suggested.

THE NON-REWARD METHOD

This method simply indicates that you withhold a reinforcement or reward if a specific behaviour is not carried out. For example: you have a contract with your child that if he takes out the garbage and mows the lawn he receives an allowance of $3.00. If he leaves the garbage and lets the grass grow, he does not get any allowance. Should you give him part of his allowance, you have reinforced an undesirable behaviour, i.e., breaking a contract. Children prefer parents to be consistent, even if they complain about the consistency.

WHAT IS PUNISHMENT?

Whether or not an act is regarded as punishment depends on the point of view and personality of the child being punished. Some children are devastated by yelling parents; others seem oblivious to verbal punishment and appear unaffected. There is some question as to whether the reaction, whatever it may be, is "learned" or is a function of the sensitivity of the child or a combination of learning and sensitivity.

Nagging, yelling, scolding, sarcasm, spanking, and the withholding of privileges are all considered punishments. Though physical punishment is used frequently by nearly 70 per cent of the more than 600 parents questioned in a recent survey, the long-term effectiveness of corporal punishment is clearly open to question. Witness, for example, the following dialogue, based on an actual interview. The problem, in this instance, was a ten-year-old boy who was smoking, lying, and still wetting his bed.

FATHER: All the methods you suggest, Doc, sound good in theory. But there's nothing that works better than a good old-fashioned whack on the ass.

H.M.: Does it really work?

FATHER: You bet.

H.M.: Then why are we discussing the problem again? Is he still smoking?

FATHER: Well, he stops for about a month, and then he forgets. All he needs is another whack and he stops again.

H.M.: Do you think if you hit him harder, or if you just keep whacking him as a reminder, that he will finally stop for good!

FATHER: You can't do that! I couldn't just hit him as a reminder.

H.M.: The test of any method of managing behaviour is whether the behaviour is eliminated, not just stopped temporarily. Physical punishment has really not worked for you, and it may have created some serious side effects – like lying, or bed-wetting. That's why we are exploring other methods to stop your son from smoking.

Physical and verbal punishment often produce quick results, but they are seldom long-lasting. In addition to their questionable effectiveness, they create negative side effects in both parent and child. In the parent, the use of punishment can leave feelings of guilt and inadequacy ("I wish I had more patience!"). On his part, the child may develop fear and anxiety, and – depending on the child's personality – punishment can produce such side effects as overaggressiveness, withdrawal, or noncomformity. Punishment also damages the child's self-esteem, and in time the youngster learns to avoid a punishing parent. It also teaches the child that hitting and yelling are acceptable "adult" ways of coping.

After working on this problem with several hundred parents, I have become convinced that there is a direct relationship between the level of an individual's parenting ability and the level of his or her use of verbal and physical punishment: the lower the level of parenting capability, the higher the use of punishment. And, as an inevitable corollary, the greater the problem with the child. As Dr. Haim Ginott has noted:

What is wrong with spanking is the lesson it demonstrates ... when you are angry – hit! Instead of displaying our ingenuity by finding civilized outlets for savage feeling, we give our children a taste of the jungle.

The most effective punishment is the *withdrawal* of privileges based on your contract with your child. You don't surprise your child with an impulsive but unjust penalty – "You were on the phone for an hour, so your phone privileges are cancelled for a month." A good family contract sets forth rules and responsibilities and spells out the consequences of infractions clearly and explicitly. There are no surprises or inconsistencies because all the ground rules have been discussed and agreed upon.

THE NEGATIVE REINFORCEMENT METHOD

Negative reinforcement differs from punishment in that the child remains in control of his or her behaviour. This allows for the termination of punishment when the child decides to end the misbehaviour. Studies of many case histories have demonstrated that whereas punishment may *stop* a given behaviour for a short period, negative reinforcement acts to *eliminate* it. One of the most effective negative reinforcers in school or at home is the *time-out procedure*.

Time-out means time away from positive reinforcers; it works best with children from three to ten years of age. The child is taken from the environment and situation in which his undesirable behaviour customarily occurs and moved to a place where there are no reinforcing people or things. There is, in short, nothing for the child to do in that new place, which might, for example, be a well-lit hallway or a bathroom.

The length of the time-out should range from three to five minutes. It must begin immediately after the inappropriate behaviour. At this point, the child is given a calm explanation of the offending act, plus a description of the consequences, and is told how he may avoid such consequences in the future. For example: "You just threw your food all over the floor. For this, you are going to stay in the hall, alone, for three minutes. If you stop throwing your food, you won't be sent out any more. *You* are in control of what happens to you."

Usually the negative behaviour decreases or is eliminated within a week if this time-out procedure is consistently, firmly, but calmly administered. "Consistently" means that the time-out follows *every time* and *immediately after* the undesirable behaviour. There is no lecturing, no screaming, no spanking – just removal from a place and situation that is reinforcing and maintaining the negative behaviour.

Experiments have demonstrated that five minutes of time out are as effective as thirty minutes. You may want to leave a kitchen timer ticking in the time-out room as an added dramatic touch. A bathroom or hallway has proven to be an effective time-out environment. However, you will want to make sure that nothing dangerous to the child is left there, and that a stay in the bathroom is really non-reinforcing (as opposed, say, to amusing or diverting).

Consider Ginny, age five. She constantly interrupts her parents' conversations and throws her food all over the table. Her parents have tried to explain to Ginny that her behaviour bothers them, and they cannot enjoy their meal when she misbehaves. They have tried paying more attention to her, but the food-throwing continues.

They decide to try time-out. Following a food-throwing incident, they firmly and without anger tell Ginny to leave the table and go into the bathroom for five minutes. They explain why this is happening and tell her she may return to the table after five minutes. There is no lecturing or reprimand, and instructions are delivered in a calm, matter-of-fact voice. Ginny screams and hollers, but mother takes her firmly into the bathroom. After five minutes she returns to the table and repeats the food-throwing. Again, gently and firmly, she is told why she is being asked to leave and for how long (again, five minutes), that she can then come back and will not be sent away again if she stops throwing her food.

The procedure takes persistence – accompanied by feelings of doubt and guilt on her parents' part – and approximately sixteen time-outs, but Ginny finally learns that the inevitable consequence could be avoided if she changes her behaviour. She stops throwing her food and – what is more – begins helping her mother to set the table, since, at the same time, her parents reinforce her positively for this appropriate behaviour.

Mickey, an excellent hockey player, was getting involved in fights in almost every game. He received numerous penalties, which cost his team several important games. His coach had warned Mickey he would bench him if he continued to fight. Mickey continued to pick fights, so the coach benched him for two games. This benching was a time-out. It took only two more benchings for Mickey to get the message and quit fighting, since he really wanted to play hockey more than he wanted to fight.

ANOTHER METHOD: REWARDING ALTERNATIVE
DESIRABLE BEHAVIOURS

This method calls for the parent to encourage and reward a behaviour directly opposed to the undesirable behaviour. In effect, the new behaviour cancels out the inappropriate one. For example, five-year-old Billy kept tearing out flowers from his father's begonia garden – Dad's pride and joy. After his father punished him, Billy pulled flowers out of a neighbour's garden. It was suggested that Dad help Billy to prepare and plant a garden of his own with an assortment of flowers. This alternative constructive behaviour was effective in eliminating Billy's destructive behaviour.

As suggested earlier, a combination of methods may, at times, be used. But the most effective, used alone or with other methods, is this last one: rewarding alternative appropriate behaviour. The focus here is not merely "How do I get rid of this obnoxious behaviour?" but, rather, "What positive acts can I encourage and reinforce that will drive out and replace the negative ones?"

Six Steps for Setting Up a Behavioural Program

Learning and unlearning are processes that flourish best with encouragement, affection, patience, practice, and strict observance of the following six steps of behaviour management:

1. Identify the specific behaviour you aim to increase or decrease.
2. Observe, count, and record the frequency of the behaviour. This forms your baseline.
3. Choose your reinforcer, and make your contract.
4. Begin to reinforce.
5. Observe, count, and record changes in the frequency of the behaviour.
6. Evaluate and (if necessary) modify.

STEP 1: IDENTIFY THE SPECIFIC BEHAVIOUR

If you say "George is bad," that's not a behaviour. It's an evaluation. It is much too vague. Be specific; pinpoint and describe the offending acts. Example: George is always hitting others. Or: George spits at other kids. Or: George grabs his friends' (brother's, sister's) toys. These are observable behaviours that you can count and record.

Another example: "Priscilla is the messiest teen-ager." This is another evaluation. Identify and pinpoint Priscilla's specific acts that you consider messy.

- She drops her clothes on the floor in every room in the house.
- Priscilla's books are all over the house.
- When she takes a bath, she leaves water on the bathroom floor, three wet towels on the floor, and her fourteen make-up jars all over the bathroom.
- Priscilla always leaves a dirty ring around the bathtub.

These are specific behaviours which, added up, characterize her as "the messiest teen-ager." Of the behaviours that you have identified, *select one* to focus on changing.

STEP 2: OBSERVE, COUNT, AND RECORD THE FREQUENCY

This will give you your *baseline*. To establish a baseline, count the number of times the behaviour occurs during a five-to-seven-day period. Both parents should attempt to count the behaviour, since a double check will give you a more reliable baseline. Perhaps you can divide the day into "shifts" during which each of you will be responsible for counting. The counting and recording are critical. Sometimes the true frequency of a given behaviour is much lower than one might have imagined it to be. It is also important to be clear on definitions. For example, what does each of you consider the elements of, say, a temper tantrum? Perhaps each parent should list these elements, in writing. The two lists can then be compared and an agreement reached so there will be accuracy in your observations and counting.

In addition to counting, you should note *when, where*, and *why* the behaviour occurred. Was there any apparent antecedent or cause for the behaviour? For example, did George hit Jimmy because George didn't know the rules of the game and couldn't play, and thus felt frustrated? These are important data.

Information from the behaviour chart gives you your baseline. Assume that you find that Peter had thirty-eight tantrums in seven days, with an average of 5.4 per day. You could graph these baseline data, as a

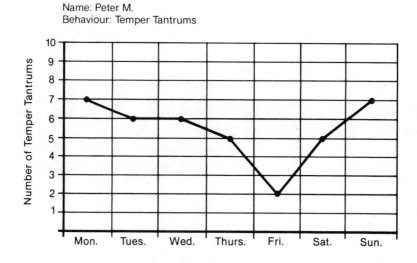

Behaviour	Mon.	Tues.	Wed.	Thurs.	Fri.	Sat.	Sun.
Temper Tantrums	⁙ll	⁙l	⁙l	⁙	ll	⁙	⁙ll
Time Interval							

Behaviour Chart

Date: Oct. 14-21

Name: Peter M.   Observer: J.M. R.M.

Where does it occur?

When does it occur?

Any cause?

Figure 13. Behaviour Chart

Behaviour Graph

Name: Peter M.
Behaviour: Temper Tantrums

Figure 14. Behaviour Graph

graph will give you a sharp picture of the behaviour during the week under study and will highlight any trends. Behaviour is customarily recorded on the vertical axis, and the time (days) on the horizontal.

If you must record for fewer hours on any given day, you can

154

establish a "rate" of behaviour for the shorter period by dividing the number of hours into the number of behaviours observed. In this manner you can, for example, compare an eight-hour observation period with one of twelve hours.

The goal, in the case involving temper tantrums, is to decrease slowly the number of tantrums per day over a period of time until they are eliminated. While collecting data, avoid nagging, yelling, spanking, or other interference with the child's behaviour. Be strict in your counting – record *all* occurrences. The behaviour chart is merely a sample, which you can modify to meet your special needs by adding space for more information, or otherwise changing. Incidentally, a golf-stroke counter is an excellent device for recording behaviours.

Be sure to explain to your child what is going on. Even if the youngster objects, carry on without apology or hesitation. Sometimes a behaviour will decrease because it is being observed. But such a fall-off will last for only a short time; the behaviour will then resume its usual frequency.

STEP 3: CHOOSE YOUR REINFORCER; MAKE YOUR CONTRACT

As recommended in the section on reinforcers, select one that is highly meaningful to your child. It should be something easy to come up with and something the youngster really wants, and it should also be within reason. Which reinforcers are within reason depends, naturally, on a family's economic circumstances, lifestyle, and values.

The probability of success is heightened if your child is involved in and excited about the contract. In the case of an older child, it is important that the child participate in the negotiations and the final agreement. With younger children, parents can make decisions unilaterally regarding the desired change and the consequent reward. Whatever the child's age, there should be a complete explanation of the reasons for the contract and of its terms. As indicated earlier, the contract should be written out and posted.

SAMPLE CONTRACTS

The following are two sample contracts. One was designed for Peter, aimed at decreasing, then eliminating, his temper tantrums (averaging 5.4 per day at the outset). For Priscilla, the challenge is cleaning up the bathroom after her bath, with its welter of wet spots, wet towels, tub rings, and cosmetic jars.

Peter (age 4½ years). Peter's temper tantrums have been increasing in frequency for almost a year. Though his parents have tried reasoning, attention-giving, scolding, spanking, ignoring, and a complete medical exam, the tantrums continue to mount. For Peter, the tantrum has become a well-learned behaviour, and almost any frustration sets it off.

The parents decided to try a behaviour management program. It was agreed by the parents that, for purposes of the program, a temper tantrum was any one or all of the following behaviours, observed by his mother and father over a long period: (1) running around the house or yard while screaming; (2) throwing objects; (3) kicking furniture, doors, or his younger brother; (4) tearing up his books, breaking his or his brother's toys. It was agreed further that, to qualify as a tantrum, the behaviour would need to continue for a minimum of one minute. The usual duration of Peter's behaviour had been one to five minutes.

The reinforcer selected was a promised visit to the Science Centre, followed by a dinner of Peter's choice at McDonald's. This prospect really excited the youngster. He was then told he would need to earn fifty poker chips (tokens) to get his reward. Since four-and-a-half-year-olds need more immediate tangible reinforcement than older children do, it was decided that Peter would receive an added bonus apart from the trip to the Science Centre and the hamburger dinner. Peter would also get an extra half hour of TV, or an extra bedtime story, for every five poker chips he earned.

The contract was carefully explained to Peter, and he was shown the behaviour chart. Peter was informed that if he had five or more tantrums in a day, he would not get any tokens at all. If he decreased the number of tantrums to four a day, he would get two poker chips. If he lowered the number to three a day, his reward would be five chips, and seven if he lowered the level to one per day. However, if he had no tantrums at all, he would get ten tokens a day.

Peter agreed to the contract. It was then written out (two copies) on the behaviour chart, with one copy posted in his room, the other on the refrigerator door. What Peter needed was a "starter," something to catalyze his change in behaviour. This contract was designed to provide that motivator, thus initiating the change.

While this contract was specifically designed to decrease and, eventually, to end a negative behaviour, it also gives his parents an opportunity to reinforce more positive behaviours as alternates to the negative. When Peter becomes frustrated and a tantrum ensues, the parents can ask themselves: How else could Peter deal with this problem? What are the child's alternatives?

It is assumed that the parents will observe and record the causes of their child's temper tantrums, the events that apparently set off the tantrums, when they occurred, and where. These concrete baseline data will prove invaluable to the parents in setting up a program to develop alternative, more productive behaviour.

At the time the tokens (poker chips) are being dispersed, the parents

Behaviour Contract

Name: Peter (age 4 1/2 years)
Goal: to stop temper tantrums

	Mon.	Tues.	Wed.	Thurs.	Fri.	Sat.	Sun.
Week 1							
Week 2							
Week 3							
Week 4							
Week 5							

Contract: 5 temper tantrums or more — 0 poker chips
4 temper tantrums — 2 poker chips
3 temper tantrums — 5 poker chips
1 temper tantrum — 7 poker chips
0 temper tantrums — 10 poker chips

For 50 poker chips, Peter gets a trip to the Science Centre, a Big Mac, and a milkshake.
For every 5 poker chips - 1/2 hour of TV or an extra bedtime story.

Figure 15. Behaviour Contract

can also award social reinforcers to show how pleased they are with the child's progress – praise, a hug, a smile, encouraging words ... recognition in any form. Social reinforcers are enormously meaningful to children. And to adults. Everyone, of whatever age, likes to be recognized and praised for his succcesses, however small.

Priscilla (age 14). In line with the six steps for setting up a behavioural program, the following steps were followed in the scenario involving Priscilla. *First,* the specific behaviour targeted for Priscilla is the bathroom mess. Priscilla is capable of changing all of these behaviours (the wet towels on the floor, the bathtub ring, and all the rest). Her parents have tried nagging, yelling, and degrading remarks, with some short-term success but with long-term failure. Constant references to Priscilla's messiness have created an unpleasant climate in the house, with limited communication between parents and teen-ager marked by anger and hostility. (Priscilla: Will I ever be glad to get out of this institution! Dad: Let me help you pack!)

Second, the frequency of the behaviour was observed, counted, and recorded for four weeks. Then, *third,* a contract was discussed and its terms agreed upon. Two reinforcers seem equally attractive to Priscilla. She has wanted for some time to invite her girl friends to the house for a barbecue, followed by a pajama party. She would also very much like to visit her favourite aunt in Washington. A point system was devised,

157

stating that if she earned 100 points she could have her barbecue and pajama party; if she earned 300 points, she could have the trip to Washington. Priscilla decided on the trip. The goals of the behaviour contract were (1) no wet towels on the floor; (2) no wet floors after the bath; (3) bathtub rings to be cleaned; (4) jars, bottles, and tubes to be put away.

Behaviour Contract

Name: Priscilla (age 14)
Goal: to clean up bathroom after bath
Consequence: +10 points for all four goals being fulfilled
             – 5 points for not fulfilling all four goals
            300 points for a 5-day trip to Washington

	Mon.	Tues.	Wed.	Thurs.	Fri.	Sat.	Sun.	Total
Week 1								
Week 2								
Week 3								
Week 4								
Week 5								
Week 6								
Week 7								
Week 8								
Week 9								

Figure 16. Behaviour Contract

The contract also specifies that there shall be no more than one bath per day (for health and economic reasons). Furthermore, Priscilla agrees that failure to live up to the contract's terms on any given day will cost her the loss of five points. During Week 1, the learning period, there will be no deductions. Her parents decide, privately, that in addition to the specified rewards, social reinforcers will be liberally awarded. Also, Priscilla and her mother will shop for new wallpaper and more attractive towels for the bathroom.

Once the contract is in effect, the *fourth step* in the behavioural program is pursued diligently by the parents. Thus, Priscilla's parents begin reinforcement immediately after every bath, without nagging or scolding because they have their end of the bargain to live up to, and verbal punishment is not in the contract. If Priscilla backslides, she loses five points for every infraction. The agreement including these terms has been written out, signed, and posted.

Concurrent with the reinforcement, the parents follow the *fifth step* as they observe, count, *and record* immediately. In addition to the behaviour chart, a behaviour graph has been drawn, by Priscilla herself, on which she will record the ups and downs in the frequency of her own behaviour. This graph provides all parties with a dramatic and powerful picture of Priscilla's progress – or lack of it.

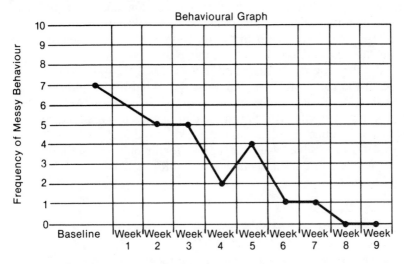

Figure 17. Behaviour Graph

From time to time, Priscilla and her parents sit down together to discuss the arrangement. Is the contract clear? Are the reinforcers still meaningful? Does the contract require modification? If the contract isn't working, perhaps different terms and rewards should be developed. This is the *sixth step*, in which the parties to the contract *evaluate and modify* it, if modification seems necessary.

Circumstances may suggest changes in the contract's terms and in the reinforcers. Assume, for example, that Priscilla suddenly becomes romantically involved with the boy next door – head over heels in love and never wanting to be apart. The reinforcers originally considered so attractive may now lose their appeal to Priscilla. After all, why should she go to Washington when she would much rather stay home, next to *him*. And who wants a bunch of giggling girls around for a pajama party, with *him* next door?

Once more, the bathroom becomes a disaster area, complete with puddles, wet towels, tub rings, and messy lotion bottles. A new contract and a different reinforcer are negotiated. The revised reinforcer: approval for a ten-minute phone session once a day (ten points), and an 11 p.m. curfew date once a week (forty points). (An observation in passing: the reinforcement chosen and agreed upon should always be reasonably flexible, in addition to being fair and meaningful.)

The Peter and Priscilla examples – based, by the way, on real-life histories – suggest certain guidelines for the development of a behaviour modification program. In each instance, the basics for a workable contract and the various steps for its implemention have been outlined. But this is, admittedly, only an outline. How it is filled in and finalized, in your case, must be determined by you and your family, based on your private circumstances, your values, and your expectations.

Were the procedures suggested in these cases the only ones appropriate to the cases of Peter and Priscilla? What about the time-out procedure, negative reinforcement, ignoring, or satiation? Would they have been just as effective? Given the complexity of human behaviour and the wide range of individual needs, skills, and background circumstances, it is impossible – even dangerous – for anyone to prescribe rigidly a *specific* procedure for *all* behaviours and for *all* children.

Limitations of Behaviour Management

Though behaviour management is a powerful and proven procedure, it has its limitations. The system may fail, or fall short, for any one of the following reasons:

1. *The child is not ready.* A young child may not be ready, in terms of his stage of development, to learn a specific behaviour. He may be limited by his intellectual, physical, or emotional capacity. Some children may never develop the capacity to learn certain behaviours.

2. *Unreal expectations.* Some parents are high achievers, and they may expect their children to reach the same level of achievement they have reached. Parents who, for example, passionately admire the music of Bach may try to develop a similar interest in a child who prefers Willie Nelson and country music. Strict religious convictions (to cite another example) may also create incompatibilities if efforts are made to develop, in the child, behaviours which conform unswervingly to the parents' convictions, especially if the child does not hold the same convictions. Such convictions will almost certainly clash head-on with those held by your adolescent's peer group. Examples: no dating before age eighteen; no premarital sexual involvements.

3. *Reinforcements may prove specific, not generic.* Reinforcement may not be a useful technique for producing *general* changes in behav-

iour as opposed to a change in one *specific* behaviour. For example, studies have shown that, in trying to reinforce young children's sharing habits and encouraging them to be generous, children may share in one *specific* training situation (after rewards are applied) but will not share in another situation. A number of theorists believe this is because these children just do not have the ability at that stage of understanding to behave in an altruistic manner. Only when they reach a more advanced level of intellectual, social, and moral understanding do they begin to develop altruistic behaviour and not need extrinsic rewards – or even social reinforcers – to do so.

True sharing or altruism, by definition, is a moral act performed voluntarily, and is an end in itself that benefits someone without any expectation of external rewards by the doer of the act. *No reinforcement schedule can develop altruism.* A child must advance through a series of stages in her/his moral development until she/he finally reaches the stage in which there is genuine sharing (altruism), usually at the age of ten to twelve years. Studies of these stages suggest that younger children (ages four to eight) will perform helping acts under certain reinforcement conditions, even though they may not yet be "truly altruistic." However, even such limited development is important, because they are thus learning how to share and how to fit into society. They are also learning the laws of reciprocity which operate in our society.

4. *Logistic weaknesses.* Other limitations of behaviour management may include weaknesses arising from unclear goals, inadequate skills, impatience, inconsistency, or lack of control over the reinforcers that are meaningful to the child.

5. *Special behaviour problems.* Certain serious behaviour problems may be more appropriately assessed and treated by a trained professional, who might prescribe specific psychotherapeutic procedures.

6. *Your patience, persistence, and consistency.* According to Ogden Lindsley, a professor of education at the University of Kansas who has conducted many behaviour modification classes for parents, it is important "if at first you don't succeed, try, try again." The majority of parents will be successful while the minority (perhaps 10 to 30 per cent) may have to try again with *smaller* goals and *different* reinforcers. Profesor Lindsley suggests that if all the steps of the behavioural program are followed, there is a 95 to 100 per cent probability of success.

Summary

In dealing with problems of juvenile behaviour, parents need access to a repertory of alternatives, such as those outlined here. And they must develop a "feel" for which procedure will be appropriate to the immediate problem.

The alternatives outlined in this chapter have been derived from learning theory and from thousands of applied research studies. But these contributions from the *science* of human behaviour management cannot be effectively applied unless they are coupled with the *art* of human behaviour. How, for example, does one measure your faith, your acceptance, and your love for your children? Love has a quality and a quantity beyond measurement by any means, scientific or otherwise. No words are adequate to define your feelings of love and caring, nor are there yardsticks to measure these feelings. But your love is there, and it exerts an enormous effect on your behaviour, your children's behaviour, and your and their relationships and growth.

Acknowledgement of the existence of love as a special dimension does not detract from the value and usefulness of the lessons we have learned about behaviour management. Awareness of the powerful role of both should emphasize, however, the need for a marriage of the two: the art of loving and caring with the science of behaviour management.

Finally, for the most effective outcome, parent-child goal setting is the ideal arrangement. And when the child or adolescent becomes the principal agent in the choice of goal and the contingencies, the probability that the goal will be achieved is maximized and he or she begins to own the responsibility for his or her motivation and behaviour.

Sample A: Behaviour Chart

Behaviour Chart

Name:
Date:
Observer:

Behaviour	Mon.	Tues.	Wed.	Thurs.	Fri.	Sat.	Sun.
Time Interval							

Where does it occur?
When does it occur?
Any cause?

Sample B: Behaviour Graph

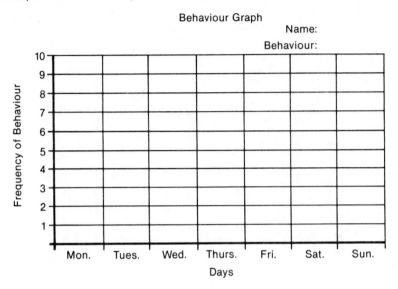

Behaviour Graph

Name:

Behaviour:

Sample C: Behaviour Graph

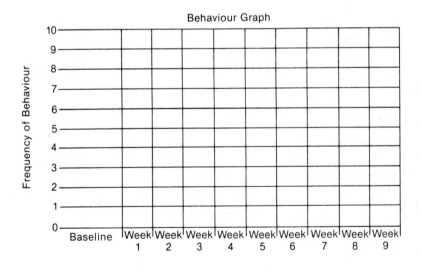

163

Sample D: Behaviour Contract

Behaviour Contract

Name:
Goal:

	Mon.	Tues.	Wed.	Thurs.	Fri.	Sat.	Sun.
Week 1							
Week 2							
Week 3							
Week 4							
Week 5							

Contract:

Sample E: Behaviour Contract

Behaviour Contract

Consequence:

	Mon.	Tues.	Wed.	Thurs.	Fri.	Sat.	Sun.	Total
Week 1								
Week 2								
Week 3								
Week 4								
Week 5								
Week 6								
Week 7								
Week 8								
Week 9								

TEN

Oh Lord, Give Me Patience!

Life creates enough hurdles – lack of patience only creates more!

Patience and Impatience

"Being a parent is not easy! What additional skills do you feel you need to cope with the problems of parenthood?" This was question twelve in our parent survey and 80 per cent of the parents answered "Patience, I need patience." There were other responses, such as understanding, insight, communication skills, a sense of humour, endurance, self-assurance, parent education, empathy, the ability to teach, to motivate, time management, good judgement, love, and forgiveness, but the predominant plea was *"I need patience."*

Interestingly enough, psychology and child psychology books do not include any mention of patience, of theories of patience, or studies of patience. Even parenting books ignore it. It's as if this human characteristic did not exist. On further investigation, I found the closest topic that was related to patience was "tolerance for frustration." For our purposes we will assume that frustration tolerance and patience are synonymous.

At first I was not sure what parents meant by "I need patience," and so I conducted a number of parent interviews and asked them "What do you mean by patience?" They referred to patience as if it was an ability or an inherited personality trait. "You are born with patience or without it." On the basis of our survey, it would appear that 80 per cent of parents are born with little of this desired and necessary trait!

In further questions, I discovered that when they said they were impatient it was a negative evaluation of their behaviour. They didn't like the way they reacted to their children's behaviour. For example:

Child's Behaviour	Parent's Behaviour	Parent's Evaluation
When Mary doesn't help with the dishes	I *nag* her.	I wish I had more patience!
When Peter plays around with his food	I *force* him to eat it.	I wish I had more patience!
When Lloyd tracks mud into the living room	I *slap* him.	I wish I had more patience!
When John moves too slowly	I *push* him.	I wish I had more patience!
When Steve takes forever to do his homework	I *yell* at him.	I wish I had more patience!
When Ed wets his bed	I *insult* him.	I wish I had more patience!
Those kids physically and mentally exhaust me so	I *eat*, I *overeat*, or I *yell* at my husband.	I wish I had more patience!
If Dorothy doesn't say "thank you" or is rude	I *pinch* her or give her a dirty look.	I wish I had more patience!
When Albert disagrees with me	I send him *to his room* without supper.	I wish I had more patience!

What parents were saying is that "I wish I didn't act that way. I wish I didn't nag, slap, push, pinch, or insult my kids." They attributed this behaviour to a lack of this special quality – patience.

WHAT IS PATIENCE?

What are its characteristics? Is it inherited or learned? How does it develop? What are the causes of impatience? Is a lack of patience all bad? How do I improve it? According to dictionary definitions, patience means to endure; to suffer calmly without complaint; not to be hasty or impetuous; to be tolerant. This chapter will attempt to take the suffering out of patience.

CHARACTERISTICS OF PATIENCE

An understanding of the concept of "threshold levels" is important to an understanding of patience. A threshold level is that "firing point" at which you become aroused or upset due to an annoyance or provocation; it is the point at which you react. Some persons have a very low patience threshold. These are easily frustrated or provoked to anger and are quick to react and strike out in almost every instance. Others, more fortunate, have a very high patience threshold. Such persons will tolerate massive doses of frustration, provocation, or personal disaster before they lose their cool.

Most of us are located somewhere between the peaks and valleys and will lose our patience only in certain circumstances. Studies have determined that different individuals are differentially vulnerable to varying kinds of annoyances. A crying baby, for example, will immediately irritate some people while leaving others undisturbed. Research results suggest that not only must a stimulant be of a given *intensity* to provoke impatience in a given individual, but it must also be of a given *kind* to excite 'hat effect in the same individual.

WHEN DO GREEN LIGHTS TURN RED?

Is patience, then, a personality trait that determines what your behaviour will be in *every* situation? No, but it determines your behaviour in *most* situations. Patience also depends on your emotional and physical state and the nature of the situation. Depending on the individual's patience threshold, he or she tends to fit into one of three broad categories: high, moderate, or low. In Figure 18, I have chosen to term individuals in these arbitrary categories as "green-light, yellow-light, and red-light" parents.

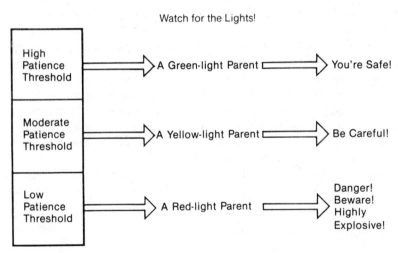

Watch for the Lights!

Figure 18. Patience Thresholds

Is a red-light parent provoked to "blow" by every situation? No. But a red-light parent is the most susceptible, the most inclined to lose his or her cool in the largest number of provocative situations. Does this mean that a green-lighter is never impatient? No. But a green-light parent "blows" rarely; it usually takes a combination of frustrating experiences to shift a green to a yellow or red.

167

For example, John is a *red-light* parent. He becomes impatient and explodes in traffic jams, waiting in restaurants, for elevators, for telephone operators, for his mail, with his mistakes, and especially with his two-year-old's crying, his four-year-old's fears, and his six-year-old's constant questions. Yet, oddly enough, Mr. Red Light may have all the patience in the world when he fishes, plays bridge, or tends his garden.

Shirley, on the other hand, is a *green-light* parent and it takes a great build-up of frustration on top of frustration before she fires off. This morning, the toaster didn't work, someone drank all the milk before breakfast, Cheryl was late for school, Terry forgot his lunch, there was a second notice of an overdue telephone bill that had been paid, and, finally, her dentist called to tell her that her appointment was cancelled after she had arranged a babysitter. She seemed to cope with all these frustrations until Terry came home from school, slammed the door, and dropped his books. Terry hit her threshold button and was the sad recipient of all the accumulated frustrations. It took the *sum* of all these frustrations to reach her threshold, i.e., her firing point. Shirley was sorry for her anger, for her yelling, for her lack of patience. *Green lights can turn red.*

From our findings it seems that the unfortunate recipients and objects of impatience are mostly our children. Children have often wished that their parents had as much patience for them as they had for their friends. *Please "treat me like you treat your friends" is a thought many kids have had.*

Most children become very sensitive to their parents patience thresholds, though some may take a verbal or physical bludgeoning before they learn to recognize what behaviours set off sparks and are red-light areas. Others have difficulty learning what behaviours are red, green, or yellow and others either withdraw inside or rebel against this low patience threshold and the punishment that follows.

We generally know our threshold level and often wish it were not so low. How did I get this way? Am I coloured red forever, or can I become a yellow or a green?

IS PATIENCE INHERITED?

Does an impatient infant become an impatient child and then an impatient adult? Is this determined by our genes? Research does suggest that although there is an inherited element to our personality, our environment and our opportunities for learning determine what we become, i.e., the product is the result of an interaction between heredity and environment. However, even though most of our genetic inheritance can be modified by our environment it is important to recognize these genetic predispositions early in childhood so that we can adjust or supply the proper environment and assistance.

Careful study of the research on the genetics of personality suggests that certain personality traits are there at birth, e.g., tendencies to be introverted or extroverted, anxious or complacent, or whether one has a high need for stimulation or a low need for stimulation and change. According to Dr. Eysenck almost 50 per cent of our anxiety level is determined by our genes.

Doctors Thomas, Chess, and Birch, who studied children from infancy to late adolescence, indicate that children differ in temperament in the first weeks of life and these differences are independent of their parents' personality or care. The temperaments seemed to be constant from birth to adolescence. They identify three types of temperaments: the "easy" child, the "slow-to-warm-up" child, and the "difficult" child (for a complete description, see Chapter 2). The temperaments of the slow-to-warm-up and the difficult child at infancy both imply a low patience level and a low tolerance for frustration. They are slow to adapt to change, are easily irritated, are generally in a negative mood, and as they grow their frustrations are evidenced by terrible temper tantrums.

The description of Clem over a seven-year period, from the research of Thomas, Chess, and Birch, portrays the difficult child who may very well become the difficult, impatient adult.

Clem exemplifies a child who scored high in intensity of reaction. At four and a half months he screamed every time he was bathed, according to his parents' report. His reactions were "not discriminating – all or none." At six months during feeding he screamed "at the sight of the spoon approaching his mouth." At nine and a half months he was generally "either in a very good mood, laughing or chuckling," or else screaming. "He laughed so hard playing peekaboo he got the hiccups." At two years his parents reported: "He screams bloody murder when he's being dressed." At seven they related: "When he's frustrated, as for example when he doesn't hit a ball very far, he stomps around, his voices goes up to its highest level, his eyes get red and occasionally fill with tears. Once he went up to his room when this occurred and screamed for half an hour."

From their long-term studies, Doctors Thomas, Chess, and Birch conclude that "a child's temperament is not immutable." Though a child's temperament is there at birth, his environment can either intensify it, modify it, or almost completely change it. Their concern is that 70 per cent of the difficult children at birth developed behavioural problems, while only 18 per cent of the easy children developed any serious emotional or behavioural problems. This suggests that the environment, specifically the parental environment, was not sufficient or capable of changing the difficult child and so the impatient infant becomes the impatient adult. The final question is, if you are an impatient adult can you modify or diminish this lack of patience? Can you *learn* to be more patient? The answer is *yes*, but the change requires that you accept the following:

1. There will always be situations in your life that will provoke and irritate and make you impatient.
2. Both patience and impatience can be learned.
3. There is no instant learning; it takes time and effort to understand, to learn the skills and strategies to change impatience to patience.
4. Life is so much easier for everyone in the family and so much more productive and fulfilling in a climate of patience.
5. The learning of patience follows the same lawful process as the learning of any skill (Learning-Hope Curve, see Chapter 4).

The Learning of Impatience

This happens early in childhood and in a number of ways. If an infant shows irritation and fussiness and cries even though there is no illness and all his or her needs have been attended to, such as being fed, burped, changed, cuddled, and played with, and if mother immediately responds to these additional demands, she has reinforced this fussiness. The child learns that "All I have to do to get her attention is cry and fuss and I get immediate action – out pops the milk." (This may be the beginning of a bad habit, i.e., treating a child's neediness with food. This early learning becomes the foundation for adult overeating and overweight. Whenever we become upset, we eat and eat.)

Many parents either can't handle the cries and screams and their child's impatient behaviour or have a real need to be loved always and so there is *instantaneous* attention. Some children have a high need for attention and are impatient when they don't get it. They whine, interrupt, or act in some inappropriate way and mothers may either drop everything and pick them up or may yell at or slap the child. Both behaviours are *attending* behaviours and the children have been successful and reinforced for their impatience. Even if a mother's reaction is negative (yelling and slapping), she at least focuses on the child. It's a case of "Hate me or love me, but don't ignore me."

Impatience may also be learned from the results of aggression that often follow frustration and impatience, if the aggression pays off. "All I have to do is get impatient, aggress verbally or physically, and I get what I want."

Our culture seems to condone and cater to the impatient and to people with a low frustration tolerance with signs and messages that say:

- Instant seating – no waiting!
- Sorry to keep you waiting.
- I'll be with you in just a moment.
- Just push the button and ....
- Instant coffee to instant diets to instant burial.

A service is a good service if it is prompt and fast. If patience has to be learned our fast-food industry is not contributing to this important quality. There is a generalization to many other spheres with subsequent experiences of failure due to a lack of patience. The world of dieting is a great example. Instant weight loss claims feed into our impatience: "Lose 20 lbs. in 20 days." According to our statistics, 80-90 per cent of those who lose the twenty pounds will regain the twenty pounds. Losing weight and maintaining the weight loss can only be achieved through great patience and much learning. Instant loss leads to instant gain. Impatience here leads to failure.

Factors Affecting Patience

Though patience may be considered a personality trait and you may be labelled a patient personality or impatient personality, there are a number of factors that affect your patience level at any one moment:

1. Physical illness and fatigue can make you more vulnerable and less capable of coping with situations. They lower your threshold point so that you "fire off" sooner. If you are up all night with a crying baby or a sick child, your threshold is lower.
2. Mental and emotional distress and mental fatigue can accentuate the seriousness of any situation affecting the accuracy of your perceptions. Your reactions may then become overreactions. "You caught me on a bad day – I was very angry because my dentist took out the wrong tooth. I'm sorry if I bit your head off because you were five minutes late."
3. Financial pressures, job loss, or a failure affect your ability to be a patient parent.
4. The extent of your understanding of the stages of child development

and of your repertoire of parenting skills can affect your patience.

5. Your personal, religious, or moral values and the intensity of your conviction may determine your ability to be patient with a person or act that opposes these values. In some instances, in fact, patience itself may be one of these values.

6. Interference with your personal goals and the lack of opportunity for self-development, personal pleasure, or privacy may affect your ability to cope with your child's behaviour or misbehaviour.

7. Low self-esteem, insecurity, or damage to your self-confidence accentuates the seriousness of any problem and results in an overreaction.

8. Having a child who is mentally handicapped, physically sick or disabled, or emotionally disturbed can produce frustration, disappointment, anger, fear, and a tiredness, all of which may lower the patience threshold.

Additional causes of impatience include:

- excessively high and unrealistic expectations of a child
- dislike of children
- an unhappy marriage
- an overload of responsibility
- an aging problem
- being too much in a child's world with unsatisfied needs for adult stimulation, company, and conversation
- a noise overload

All these factors can influence how patient you are as a parent. By being aware of (a) how these factors can affect your perception of a situation, and (b) how they can lower your patience and cause you to overreact, you can better assess a situation, stay in control, and prevent the consequences of impatience.

The Stress Reactions and Consequences of Impatience

Impatience in its extreme form typifies (a) the type of personality whose impatience leads to heart attacks and (b) the child abusers whose impatience beats, bruises, and burns physically, mentally, and emotionally. Psychosomatic illnesses that result from impatience are legion and well-documented; they include ulcers, hypertension, muscle tension, headaches, dermatitis, and backaches. Impatience and a low tolerance for frustration can lead to overworking, overeating, excessive drinking, increased smoking, and drug use. Impatience can cause the alienation of others, regression to immature behaviour, and a decline in the ability to solve problems.

Impatience with children is often a transfer of impatience with another situation. For example, it may be unacceptable to be impatient with your boss but when you return home frustrated it seems acceptable to unload your impatience on your children or your spouse. Another serious consequence is that you give legitimacy to impatience because you are an adult, the person who sets the example and standards of behaviour for your children to model. They learn to react to frustration by imitating the giants in their lives – their parents. Finally, one of the most serious consequences is the cost in terms of a good parent-child relationship. The negative environment created in the home by impatience rarely accomplishes anything positive.

These are some of the factors that affect our level of patience and some of the consequences of impatience. It is not suggested that the 80 per cent of parents who wish for more patience experience all of the above, but they may find here some explanations for their impatience.

ELEVEN

The Secret to Patience:

Don't Make Everything a 10!

Stress Management Strategies

PREVENTION AND REDUCTION OF IMPATIENCE

How does one begin to improve one's patience? As most therapists agree, improvement begins with (1) a recognition of your lack of patience, (2) identification of the cause of your behaviour, (3) understanding the total process of patience, and (4) the development of strategies for the prevention or resolution of impatience and the reduction of the emotional overreaction to stressful situations.

The following five-stage model can be used to understand the process, pinpoint the problems, and help prevent impatient behaviour. It explains the sequences in the development of impatient behaviour. One stage leads to the next. The value of this model is that it can help us to zero in and make corrections in the early stages of the process and, thereby, "prevent" impatient behaviour. The goal of this model is not only to *reduce* the negative effects of impatience, but also to offer strategies that will *prevent* impatience.

THE FIVE STAGES IN THE LAMP SAGA

Stage 1: Cause or Problem. While Peter was playing in the living room, he broke your favourite lamp.

Stage 2: The Appraisal – The Rating. It's a 10! It's catastrophe! It's your favourite lamp and it's not replaceable. He's careless, inconsiderate, and bad!

Stage 3: Your Emotional Reaction. Your appraisal makes you angry. You're boiling and you go into a rage.

Stage 4: Your Physical and Verbal Reaction. In your anger you don't listen to any of his explanations. Instead, you yell at Peter, grab him, and whack his bottom.

Stage 5: Your Evaluation of Stage 4. Peter cries and runs to escape from you. You don't like the way you overreacted. You tell yourself that no lamp is more important than your son. You are not even certain he was to blame. You would never treat anyone else like that. Hitting has never solved a problem in the past. You feel *inadequate* in the way you dealt with the problem, your feelings of *guilt* lead to "I wish I had more patience!" Wishing, unfortunately, won't make it so.

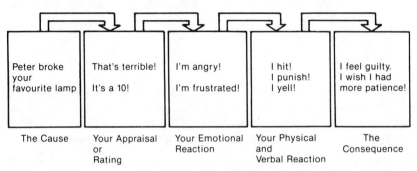

Peter broke your favourite lamp	That's terrible! It's a 10!	I'm angry! I'm frustrated!	I hit! I punish! I yell!	I feel guilty. I wish I had more patience!
The Cause	Your Appraisal or Rating	Your Emotional Reaction	Your Physical and Verbal Reaction	The Consequence

Figure 19. The Five Stages Leading to Impatient Behaviour

Intervention Strategy #1: The Cause

> Peter broke your favorite lamp.

The first intervention strategy calls for you to examine the "why" of the incident. Why and how did Peter break the lamp? A calm, reasoned answer to this question may head off all the rest of the stages. A simple check list is a good place to begin.

1. Was the lamp-breaking accidental or intentional?
2. What caused Peter to do that?
3. How frequently does this kind of behaviour occur?
4. How can you change the situation to prevent such incidents?

ACCIDENT OR INTENTION?

Did Peter break the lamp intentionally, out of anger, or accidentally? Punishment should fit the crime and our democratic system of justice takes into account whether there is intent in a misdemeanour. Unfortunately, many parents use the authoritarian system of justice. Because of their almost total control of the home environment, some parents dispense punishment based on their anger rather than on justice.

It is important to differentiate between accident and intent. As adults we accidentally break many things. There are always avoidable and unavoidable accidents involving adults as well as children. If Peter was playing ball or frisbee in the living room, the lamp breaking was an avoidable accident and one that can be avoided in the future by a strict rule: "Ball playing or frisbee is allowed in the basement or outside, but not in any other room in the house because balls and frisbees can break things or hurt people. The living room is strictly for reading, conversation, or TV watching."

CHILD-PROOFING

If you expect Peter to play in that room, child-proof it. It's not fair to place a delicate lamp in an area of active play. Physical activity is necessary for children and many homes are not considerate of this basic need. Try to design your living environment so that you provide a place to play. Children learn through play. When you restrict their play you limit their opportunities for learning. Some homes are designed for appearance and effect and not for living. Check your priorities. Good planning eliminates crisis management.

EXPECTATIONS AS A CAUSE

Unrealistic expectations and overly high standards may be at the root of your child's behaviour and the cause of his misdemeanours. He simply may be unable to meet your expectation or live up to your standards. They may be beyond his capacity.

Example. You want Doug to become a great baseball player. You chauffeur him to practice every day but he never makes the team. You're angry and impatient with him, and on the way home you criticize and insult him. Is it possible that (a) Doug doesn't want to be a ballplayer or that (b) he is neither physically nor emotionally ready for Little League?

Example. You have taken your family to a very good restaurant. Service is slow, and Karen, eight years old, begins to fidget between the soup and the main course. The conversation is adult and does not include or interest her. In her fidgeting she knocks over a crystal glass of water. The glass breaks and spills water all over your new dress. You push Karen into her seat, and with quiet, smouldering anger you hiss, "Wait until you get home. You're impossible!" No one enjoys the rest of the meal.

This situation can be avoided. The expectation that Karen can sit still for two hours in the midst of adult conversation is unfair and an imposition. To avoid the breakage of glass and relationships, select a restaurant with simple service and menu and focus your attention on Karen as well as the others. *Listen* to her. Tell her about your day's adventures and misadventures. If your expectation is that Karen will act

176

like an adult – she's not and your demands and expectations may be setting her up for some inappropriate behaviour.

TREAT THE CAUSE, NOT THE SYMPTOM

A child's negative behaviour is often a message that something is wrong and the behaviour is only a symptom. If you react only to the symptom, you may be able to prevent a repetition of that specific behaviour. But the actual cause may erupt into another negative behaviour. Treating the symptom and not the cause is like putting powder on a pimple – you may cover it up, but it is still there and festering.

Example. You are impatient with your child's eating and overweight, and you lash out with belittling comments and demeaning restrictions. The eating behaviour may be the tip of the iceberg; the hidden mass of the iceberg may be some failure, some inadequacy, or a loneliness that is provoking the overeating.

Intervention Strategy #2: Don't Rate Everything 10!

That's bad! "It's a 10!"

Your Evaluation From 1 to 10

Rate the seriousness of the behaviour on a scale from 1 to 10, where 1 is a trivial behaviour and 10 is a terrible crime, misdemeanour, or disaster. This is perhaps the *most important step* in the prevention and management of impatience since all else follows this first evaluation: your anger, your punishment, your feelings of guilt, and finally your "wish" that you have more patience.

Some parents react as if every infraction were a 10! It becomes a stylized reaction. What is a 1 for you? A 5? A 10? Breaches of courtesy could be a 1 or 2, breaches of confidence perhaps a 3. Breaches of moral behaviour the child could reasonably be expected to have mastered, a 5 or more. Disobedient behaviour with potentially serious consequences (e.g., hitting someone with an object; drug involvement), a 7 or more.

In our parent workshops, the problem of patience is always high on the agenda. Parents ask for assistance in dealing with problems patiently and we use the model described above for our analyses. Perhaps the most constructive learning experience comes when parents share their views on the rating of various behaviours. For example: How would you rate lying?

PARENT A: That's a 10! I dislike lies. They are not necessary, they really make me angry!

PARENT B: A 10? I think you're wrong. A chronic liar is serious, but even that is not a 10. I would rate it a 5, and I would really investigate why he lies so much. What's he trying to cover up?

177

PARENT C: I agree. I would probably rate chronic lying of a four-year-old a 3 or 4, but if my sixteen-year-old daughter was constantly lying, I would rate it a 6 or 7.

Parents begin to realize that you can overrate or underrate. They begin to see, too, that *overrating* is often the cause of their impatience, of their full-blown explosions, and of their later guilt and regrets. There is enormous personal cost and long-term damage to interpersonal relationships when you overreact and hit out.

Parents in the discussion groups usually change their perceptions and ratings of their children's behaviours. The ratings may move from 10's to 7's and from 7's to 4's. With this down-scaling of ratings they usually become less impatient and less angry, feel less guilty, and deal more positively and constructively with their children's behaviours. Note, however, that changing a rating from a 7 to a 3 is not being more permissive. It's being more rational in your evaluation of the seriousness of the situation.

Some husbands have claimed that their wives were exaggerating the frequency and intensity of the problem behaviour, and some wives have challenged their husbands on the same score. From these differences in perception we developed the idea of *keeping a diary*, in which their child's misdemeanours were recorded, noting when they occurred, why, and how frequently. In most cases there was a noticeable tendency to exaggerate or overestimate. This data proved extremely helpful to parents in their understanding of misbehaviours and in their planning. They learned to ask questions. Was it an accident? Did the child really understand what he was doing? This questioning began to be reflected in lower ratings. The parents began to recognize as well the reasons for their ratings and the factors that influenced a rating of 7 or 9. Questions of values of child-rearing styles often explain the 2's or 10's.

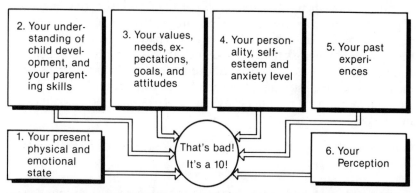

Figure 20. Factors that Affect Your Evaluation of Children's Behaviour

1. How did you feel at that moment of rating? If you're physically exhausted, if you hadn't slept all night because of pain or worry, any misbehaviour appears more serious, a 3 becomes a 5. If you are emotionally exhausted, a 4 can become a 7.

2. Your understanding of a child's capacities, abilities, readiness, and stages of development will help you to evaluate the appropriateness or inappropriateness of his or her behaviour. For example, a child of five may know some of the rules of right and wrong, but has not as yet grasped and developed a mature concept of morality or justice. Again, if you are not familiar with the normal age range of speech development you may become impatient with your two-year-old's slow but normal speech and language development because you compare him with a child at the high end of the range.

3. Your values and standards may be out of touch with current societal values or peer values. Your values will be reflected in your ratings. Conflicts over values lead to expressions of friction and impatience. Similarly, your needs and expectations may or may not be appropriate to your child's needs or his abilities and thus in your eyes what otherwise might be about a 4 behaviour becomes an 8.

4. If you have a low self-concept and feel inadequate you will tolerate less. If you have an anxious personality your ratings will reflect this. Some parents are bothered by too much stimulation and so become impatient. Your perceptual ability is a factor, i.e., your interpretation of what you see may not be accurate. Impulsiveness may also affect your ratings. Your personality is a critical factor in your evaluation and it must be considered.

5. If you have had some experience with children's behaviours, it gives you some direction as to what interpersonal techniques worked and didn't work in the past and also it puts a particular behaviour into a total perspective.

6. Your perception of a behaviour is your personal interpretation, which is based on your past experience. Perception is not always an 'exact duplicate of what is actually there. So there can be wide individual differences between perception and reality. Perception is also affected by the other five factors.

It's important to be aware of these factors if you wish to understand your evaluation and your impatience. When you consider the possible factors that influence your rating, your 10's can become 3's and this reduces your anger and the behaviour that you label as impatient. You will like yourself and Peter better.

Stopping briefly in the heat of the moment to check your rating is a powerful *preventative* procedure when you are about to punish a child. In addition to assisting you in the development of patience, it's an important lesson to teach children. They also live with and suffer from impatience. You can't legislate their appraisal, but by sharing and comparing the *why* of your ratings, you can help them develop more realistic judgements.

Intervention Strategy #3: Check Your Emotional Reaction

> I'm irritated!
> I'm angry!
> I'm frustrated!

Your appraisal and your rating of your child's misbehaviour lead to an emotional response that could be anger, hostility, or frustration. The higher you rate the seriousness of the behaviour, the greater the emotional reaction and the greater the cost to your system. If you have a low frustration threshold, fire off easily, and rate every behaviour a 10, your anger can create muscular tension which, in turn, affects your neuro-endocrine system and the automatic nervous system, causes spasms in the digestive tract, and constricts the muscles of the arteries. This physiological upset can then be responsible for headaches, backaches, ulcers, high blood pressure, and many other psychosomatic illnesses. These in turn affect your mental state and your performance and relationships at home or on the job. 10's are costly. Generally your ratings are directly related to your emotional response. Does this mean one should never get angry? No! But if 80 per cent of the parents wish desperately for more patience, this indicates that they are becoming overly emotional, are overreacting, and are paying for it.

THE RIGHT TO ANGER

You have the right to become angry when, after two explanations and three warnings, David still persists in leaving the freezer door open and the hot water tap running. Some parents try hard to be popular with their children at all times and so repress and hide their anger. Others pride themselves on "My kids have never seen me upset or angry." This is not a healthy popularity or a healthy pride. Repressed anger has to come out somewhere and often it comes out inappropriately. Parents have the right to anger and children have the right to be made aware of their parents' anger.

One of the most informative books on childhood is Carole Klein's *How It Feels To Be A Child*. Every parent should read it to understand childhood and adolescence. Her central message is that if we don't want our children to become emotional cripples, they should have the right to experience the entire range of emotions – fear, loneliness, anger, anxiety, joy, pride, and all the rest. If children are to cope with the many difficult and painful realities of life, they must not be protected from these emotions. The human system, according to Klein, is built to withstand "emotional bruising," and maturity comes from the experiencing of these feelings. Identifying and acknowledging them are important in each individual's growing process.

Klein debunks the myth of the forever-happy child, which encourages children to deny too much of the reality in human experience. Efforts by parents to keep their children always happy and to cushion their feelings of anger and of loneliness stunt their emotional growth. How can you deal with anger as an adult if you have never learned how to deal with it as a child? If a child's only perception of life is that it is "sugar and spice and everything nice," adult reality will be too much to cope with. According to Klein, the feeling of anger should not bring guilt. *What you do about your anger may justify guilt.* The feeling of anger has been built into the human system and serves a purpose. It alerts, it prepares, it energizes; it sends messages that say "I hurt," "I'm upset," "I'm concerned," or "I care." To submerge anger, to deny it, to repress it and not deal with it can lead to serious problems.

The acknowledgement of the legitimacy of anger is related to patience. If we have a feeling of guilt because of our feeling of anger, we become more impatient with this perceived weakness. If we try to bottle it up, it builds and builds and then explodes with more anger than the situation calls for. This then leads to more primitive, punitive reactions and to our concern for our lack of patience. To prevent this from happening, if your child's behaviour gets a rating of 5 to 10, let yourself be angry. It's a legitimate, normal emotion. Dealing positively and constructively with a situation reduces anger, whereas negative action increases anger and guilt. Anger that cannot be translated into positive, constructive reaction is like a hurricane and destroys whatever is in its path.

The amount of anger should be related to your rating system. That is why it's important to appraise and rate your child's behaviour realistically. However, there will be times when your intellectual appraisal of the behaviour is a 3, but your emotions register a 7 for you. This imbalance may result from any one of the many factors that affect your appraisal of the situation, e.g., your present emotional or physical fatigue or your anxious personality. You know you shouldn't feel this way; you know why you feel this way; and yet the anger or anxiety is there. What can you do about it?

Research has clearly demonstrated that a certain level of emotion can actually improve your performance. It mobilizes and energizes. However, too much emotion debilitates, that is, it can damage your effectiveness in coping with a task or problem. On the basis of our past history, most of us are aware when we are too anxious, but few of us have learned a method of *stress reduction* that will bring our anger and anxiety down to a level where it is not harmful to us or others.

You not only have to check your evaluation of a situation that makes you upset and impatient, but you need to have a strategy or a repertoire of strategies to reduce the anger or anxiety if it should build up. Often it's not just one incident that causes impatience, but a build-up of events such as an argument at work, being overlooked for a promotion, the runaway cost of living, overdue bills, a dent in your rear fender, and your wife's sister (a two-pack-a-day smoker) who is visiting for a month. There is an accumulation of anxiety, fear, frustration, and anger. There is acid in your gastrointestinal system and acid in your treatment of anything that gets in your way. Unfortunately, the smallest, the youngest, the weakest often bear the brunt.

Johnny (age 7) thought he would help Dad by washing and polishing his car. He used a floor wax that took the finish off. When Dad discovered the splotches on the car, he took the finish off little Johnny. All the pressure from that seething cauldron of emotion burst and Johnny was in the way. When the storm blew itself out, Johnny, the victim, lay crying in his room, his bottom hurt, his pride hurt. He was confused and angry and thoughts ran to hate and revenge. The relief for Dad was momentary; he felt guilty – *"I wish I had more patience!"* He had not resolved any of the causes of his anger, frustration, and stress; he only added some guilt for victimizing someone he loved so much.

Parents live in a world of pressures and concerns. These are inevitable and will always be part of the human condition. We need strategies to *prevent* and *reduce* and *resolve* the pressure.

Stress Management Procedures

1. *Prevention*
   A. Identify the *stressor* (i.e., what's bothering you).
   B. Check your perception or interpretation of the stressor. (Are you reading the situation correctly?)
   C. Check your rating of the importance of the stressor or incident. (Is it a 1 or a 10?)
   D. Check out all the factors that influence your perception and rating of a stressor. (Are they the *real* cause of your stress and impatience?)
2. *Reduction*
   A. Identify your emotional reaction and recognize how it affects you physically and mentally.
   B. If you overreact emotionally to pressure, develop some strategies to reduce this emotionality and its negative effects.

3. *Resolution*
    Check your present problem-solving methods and your alternatives.

VENTILATION

The emotional pressure that builds up must have a safety valve or else it erupts.

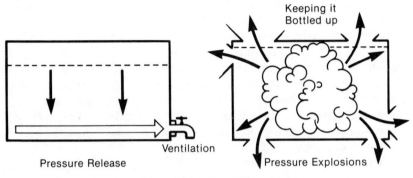

Figure 21. Ventilation of Pressure

One important safety valve is ventilation. Sharing your anxiety with your spouse, your children, a friend, a clergyman, or a therapist, "talking it out" to an empathetic, non-judgemental listener lowers the pressure and reduces negative outcomes. It can get you back into balance and into control. Solutions come more readily with less heat. All your energies are not being expended and preoccupied with your anxiety, but can instead be focused on problem-solving.

POSITIVE SELF-STATEMENTS

Much of our behaviour is determined by our expectations. Substantial research by a Harvard team of scientists demonstrates that a person's expectation serves in itself to create a self-fulfilling prophecy. Their study of the effect of teachers indicates a teacher's *expectation* of a child's intellectual performance actually determines his performance. If she thinks he's bright, even if she has not seen him perform, he ends up performing according to her expectations. Parents' behavioural expectations of themselves and their children often make that behaviour happen! Expectations are translated into self-statements, e.g., "I just know that this kid is going to give me a hard time today" or "I'm going to fail this exam" or "I probably won't be able to fall asleep tonight" or "This is going to be a great day." There are negative and positive self-statements.

A very important and successful trend in stress reduction programs centres on changing expectations and, specifically, changing the negative self-statements to positive self-statements. A self-statement is what you think or say to yourself. Thinking is internal talking to yourself. We all do it constantly and research has demonstrated that negative self-statements lead to an increase in anxiety, anger, poor performance, and negative self-fulfilling prophecies.

In questioning Olympic athletes regarding their self-statements, I have found that many who have done poorly in an event had the following self-statements: "This is not my day." "I don't feel up for this competition." "I'm going to blow it." "I'm too nervous." These athletes have been training for years and are capable of high performance, and so I have instructed them to change their negative self-statements to positive self-statements, such as: "I've done this routine on the beam successfully a hundred times. I'm going to get up and do it today!" "I'm up for it." "This anxiety is good for me, my systems are all go!" "I feel real good." "Nothing else exists right now – it's just me and that event." These positive self-statements have proven to be tremendously successful. They allow an individual to keep stress at a level that facilitates maximum performance. They are not messed up with negative doom-and-gloom self-statements.

I have recommended this same procedure for impatient parents with equal success. I had questioned many parents who felt guilty and inadequate with their lack of patience and found that there is a sequence to a parent's negative self-statements. It begins with the first self-statement: (1) *anticipating* a child's behaviour: "He's *going to* spill that juice all over the floor." With the next self-statement you are (2) *preparing* your reaction to the child's behaviour. "If he spills that I'm going to let him have it. I told him to sit at the table and drink his juice." (3) The next self-statement after he spills the juice all over the floor and you react with a slap is "This kid's impossible, he's driving me up a wall." (4) The final self-statement is "Why, oh why can't I control myself better – I'm so impatient."

Our collection of other negative parent self-statements include:

"He's never going to learn."

"Why doesn't she stop and use some common sense?"

"Why doesn't he pay attention?"

"It's his fault."

"I wonder what trouble George is going to get into next?"

"I just don't know how to handle this kid!"

"She is just trying to spite me."

These are some of the negative self-statements used before and during or

184

after a child's behaviour. They end up creating a lot of anger, heat, overreactions, and guilt.

This procedure does not suggest that when your child spills something all over the broadloom that you say to yourself, "Terrific, it's only my new broadloom and chocolate milk doesn't leave much of a stain." It does suggest that you become *aware* of the nature and frequency of these negative self-statements. The negative self-statements and negative thinking can be a general style of thinking toward yourself or others. "I can't do it" or "He can't do it" leads to anxiety and to "not doing it."

Extensive research studies have been made into the effects of negative self-statements and the effects of training procedures for changing negative to positive self-statements with children who have learning and emotional problems, with the overweight, with athletes, with individuals preparing for examinations or job interviews, and with parents. Both research and clinical reports show evidence of significant improvement as a result of individuals changing from negative to positive self-statements.

This improvement is not instantaneous. There is a procedure and a learning process. The steps in the procedure include *becoming aware* and *taking inventory* of your thinking and self-statements prior to a situation. Write them down, examine them, and begin to change as many negatives to positives as you can. For parents, this often includes changing the focus from "How do I punish this kid?" to "How can I prevent this from happening again and how do I teach him a better way?"

A Positive Self-statement

"I'm going to tell her that we all have duties and we all have privileges in this house. I work all day and I really need her help to set the table and assist with meal preparation and cleaning up."

A Negative Self-statement

"That kid is just lazy! I'm tired of having to come home, make dinner, and do the dishes. Wait 'til I see her, she's going to get a piece of my mind because I know she's going to run off without helping."

The negative self-statement is creating anxiety, tension, and acid in the gastrointestinal tract. It generally leads to yelling, nagging, insulting, slapping, and, for 80 per cent of parents, "I wish I had more patience." Take a look at your alternative positive self-statements; they generally lead to more positive reactions and positive outcomes and reduce your emotional reactions. Your mind is capable, through negative thoughts, of creating tension, anxiety, and much pain.

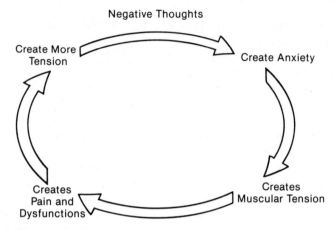

Figure 22. Negative Thoughts and Their Results

The "flip side" of this is that your mind is also capable of eliminating tension and the pain that follows.

Relaxation Procedures

A fundamental fact: you cannot be relaxed and anxious at the same time. They are two opposites like hot and cold. If you learn how to relax and are able to induce this state of relaxation when you need it, you can then reduce your level of anxiety. You are in control.

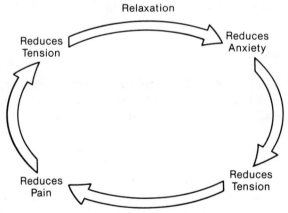

Figure 23. Relaxation and Its Results

There are a number of relaxation procedures: yoga, transcendental meditation, autogenic training, Jacobson's Muscle Relaxation, and a Breathing Muscle Relaxation method (BMR) that I have been using with Canadian Olympic athletes. Relaxation methods have proven to be extremely effective in reducing anxiety for parents, teachers, businessmen, and professionals in different stress situations. It is a learning and, like all learning, it takes time to learn and follows the Learning-Hope Curve. At first you may not feel any different, but with perseverance it becomes easier and easier to create this feeling of relaxation that reduces both psychological and physiological signs of tension.

BIOFEEDBACK

Voluminous research has proven that stress can cause serious physical illness such as heart attacks, ulcers, high blood pressure, headaches, and many other disabling medical problems. Through the work of Dr. Neil Miller of Rockefeller University and our space-age electronics it has been demonstrated that we can mentally control the tension in our musculature and in the autonomic nervous system, which in turn controls our heart rate, glandular secretions, and oxygen consumption.

The technical equipment for the research is simple. A sensor attached to the individual registers the autonomic response, e.g., heart rate, which is then translated into an auditory signal. A loud signal means a fast heart rate, a low signal indicates a slow heart rate. This is the feedback signal which the individual using relaxation can learn to voluntarily manipulate up or down and so increase or decrease his own heart rate.

This method has been successfully used in the reduction of muscle tension in the forehead and the subsequent headaches that stem from this tension. Patients with irregular heart beats, arrhythmia, have also been trained to restore normal rhythms. It has also been demonstrated that people can be trained to regulate their brain waves, which are also indicants of emotional and thinking processes. Biofeedback, like the other stress reduction methods, does not necessarily solve all your problems, but it does help to reduce excess anger and anxiety so that new problems are not created by the impatience that comes with high emotionality.

PHYSICAL ACTIVITY

Involvement in sport and physical activities serves a number of functions in the reduction of anxiety. It allows for the syphoning off of built-up energy; it's fun and exhilarating; it diverts the mind from its preoccupation with problems; it repairs and builds the physical and physiological systems which, in turn, affect the intellectual and emotional systems. In short, physical activity is a respite that clears the head and gives you a fresh perspective on your problems.

Many people report that they experience important insights during relaxation or physical activity. "It's as if all that pressure that sits on my problem-solving equipment is released." The physical activity can be a walk, a hike, tennis, jogging, dancing, touch football, fishing, or a sexual cavort.

MUSIC AND ARTS

For many individuals either playing an instrument or listening to Beethoven, Debussy, John Lennon, or Willie Nelson can have a soothing, tranquilizing effect. "Music soothes the savage breast" is more than just an adage. An involvement in painting, sculpture, woodworking, or whatever art form or hobby can also serve to reduce your level of anxiety.

HUMOUR AND LAUGHTER

It's also important to park your gloom, not take yourself too seriously, and be able to see, learn, and appreciate the humour that surrounds us. Humour is a safety valve: it allows the pressure to diminish. It can be found watching a Woody Allen movie or listening to a funny story. It may be remembering your wife turning on the blender to make the kids a milkshake without putting the cover on the blender, or when you threw the anchor out and forgot to tie it on to the boat, or getting it in the eye while changing your son's diaper. These funny situations syphon off the pressure and give our lives a special quality. We must never lose our sense of humour – it helps us to survive.

Norman Cousins, in *Anatomy of an Illness* where he documents how "one man proved your mind can cure your body," emphasizes the critical and therapeutic role of laughter and humour in his survival. "I made the joyous discovery that ten minutes of genuine belly laughter had an anesthetic effect and would give me at least two hours of pain-free sleep.... I was greatly elated by the discovery that there is a physiologic basis for the ancient theory that laughter is good medicine."

PRAYER

Whatever your religious persuasion, prayer can be a powerful safety valve. It can reduce the level of anxiety and strengthen resolve. I have seen its powerful effects when people are seriously ill, troubled, or going into a stressful performance. One cannot legislate belief, but if belief is there the expression of this belief serves to reduce tension and refurbishes one's resolve and ability to cope with stress.

DRUGS

There are situations where a physician's prescription of a sedative or tranquilizer is necessary. One's concern about the use of drugs is that this can move from a temporary emergency procedure to a permanent *habit*

188

in the control of stress. There are millions who have become dependent on and addicted to tranquilizers. This addiction does not resolve any problem. It's a momentary turn-off and prevents new learning of how to cope. There is no magic drug for patience!

LEARNING TO "PARK"

We create more problems and we become more impatient when we constantly carry our concerns around to every new situation. It becomes difficult to be effective or to enjoy the good times. To be able to cope with our everyday problems we have to learn to park them. "To park" means you're going to leave them for a while, but you will return to pick them up so that you can work on resolving them. The *parking period* allows you to focus effectively on a new task or person completely and not be preoccupied with what has happened before. It gives you time for repair of run-down, tired systems. You "park" when you go into your relaxation procedures, when you are involved in physical activity, music, or any other art form or hobby.

COUNTER-PRODUCTIVE STRATEGIES

Alcohol, overeating, and increased smoking add problems to your problems and accelerate the emotional eruption. As Shakespeare noted, "Momentary joy breeds months of pain and cold disdain."

Finally, our system is built to absorb some of the emotional build-up so that we can remain patient and in control. But in our complex, pressured society we need to learn a set of positive strategies that will reduce the emotional build-up so that there is no self-damage or damage to others. These suggested safety valves can decrease anxiety and anger and increase your coping abilities.

It's important, however, to remember that these strategies may serve to *reduce* and *siphon* off the pressure, but they do not necessarily *solve* the original cause of your anger. Their function is to add to the quality of your life and keep you in a balanced emotional state so that you can more clearly understand the problems and explore alternatives to resolve and eliminate them.

Intervention Strategy #4: Your Verbal and Physical Reaction

Stage 4	I hit! I punish! I yell! I insult!

Would you teach your child to react as follows:

	Yes	No
1. If I annoy you just yell at me!		
2. If your friends frustrate you, hit them!		
3. If your teacher irritates you, punch her!		
4. If your grandma bothers you, push her!		
5. If the minister preaches too long, insult him!		
6. Make sure you only hit someone smaller, less powerful, and dependent on you!		

Even though the causes for anger in these questions may be legitimate, the reactions are not. Obviously you would not answer yes to any of the above, and obviously 80 per cent of the parents interviewed commit these acts toward their children frequently and that's why the plea, "I need patience! I feel guilty and I don't like to react that way."

Since a child's best learning mode is by imitation and modelling, your slap teaches "when frustrated – slap! It's the adult way; it's mature behaviour." You have now given legitimacy and licence for this behaviour and this behaviour becomes an infectious style. Between 70 to 80 per cent of parents in North America use physical punishment in some situations and it probably is the same 80 per cent who would like to develop more patience with their children's behaviour.

Their dissatisfaction is more than just a function of their guilt, it's also a recognition that the behaviour doesn't correct or doesn't eliminate the inappropriate behaviour. It may terminate it and submerge it for a short period, but eventually it reoccurs.

WHEN IS PUNISHMENT CHILD ABUSE?

By virtue of your size, control, and power, you are able to punish your child verbally, physically, and emotionally. Many parents take advantage of this power position. Is this child abuse? We think of child abuse as a specific pathology, an illness, but when does your verbal, emotional, and physical punishment become abuse? Is there a difference between a child abuser who, in a rage, injures his child by breaking his arm and the parent who, in a rage, slaps his child on the bottom or across the face? Are both abusers? When is hitting, insult, withdrawal of affection, or yelling not abuse? We are beginning to acknowledge that it is a dimensional problem and that, if our society condones a little child abuse, it sets the scene and gives licence for the severe child abuse.

It's encouraging that parents are saying, "I wish I had patience," because this is the first step in the realization that there must be another way. The only concern is that some parents feel that their patience level is inherited, fixed, and immutable when we know that it can be changed by learning alternative methods to cope with frustrations.

WHAT ARE THE ALTERNATIVES?

Parents need to learn alternatives to deal with a child's behaviour in a more professional and reasonable manner. "Professional" means skilfully and effectively. You have the right to feel angry, but not the right to be preoccupied with this anger. When a surgeon operates we expect him or her to have some feeling and concern, but if something goes wrong we expect the surgeon to be preoccupied with problem-solving and not with personal feelings. We expect this professional approach from our children's teachers, who have to deal with a class of thirty very different individuals. In any one class the teacher may have three kids talking, two fighting, two daydreaming, one picking his nose, one with a bladder problem, and one constantly interrupting. We do not expect or accept a teacher's behaviour that includes yelling, pushing, hitting, or insults. We expect her or him to keep cool, to be in control, and to resolve the problems with expertise and not hysteria.

I sit in awe of elementary and high school teachers and their problems of the individual differences in learning styles, learning rates, motivation, attention, and self-control. Teachers have an overwhelming task and the more skilful are the more patient. And that is the essence of patience – skill and understanding. The alternatives begin with: (1) an *understanding* of the stages of patience, i.e., how impatience develops; (2) an *awareness* of your patience threshold level, i.e., whether you are quick-tempered with a short fuse or are slow to anger; (3) an *acknowledgement* that, (a) I don't know how else to handle the problem; (b) I'm tired; (c) I'm in an anxious state; (d) I am a perfectionist; or (e) I just don't understand kids.

These preliminary acknowledgements are important since they may explain the *why* of your impatience and begin to give you some direction for improvement. A number of other alternatives should be considered next.

(4) Check to see whether the problem is the child's behaviour or an impatience and frustration that you bring to the situation. If it is the latter, deal with this before you vent your impatience on the unsuspecting. If, at the end of a difficult day, you come home frustrated, irritated, and ready to blow, try to share this with your family. This will alert them and give them understanding. Your ventilation itself helps you release the emotional pressure and you will probably get the support you need at that moment. That's what a family is for. It should be a harbour of love, acceptance, and unequivocal support. "I'm so tired and upset, my secretary quit, a customer cancelled a large order, my sales manager

blasted me, and I left the lights in my car on all day!" Depending on how it is resolved, this background can either lead to big trouble or to an easing of the pain.

(5) Check out the "why" of your child's behaviour. As indicated earlier, treat the cause not just the symptom. For example, if Tony comes home from school and punches his younger brother, this behaviour is unacceptable. It is important to deal with the punch, but it is also important to investigate the background of the punch. Tony failed his math and reading again today; his teacher embarrassed him in front of the class and his friends teased him on the way home. It was a rotten day and he vented his frustration on the first person he encountered, his little brother, Jimmy, who was a vulnerable target for his anger. Tony needed some help to deal with his failures. He needed patience, empathy, and direction from his parents and perhaps help from a tutor. Reacting to the punch alone does not correct the problem. Tony may stop hitting Jimmy but the built-up frustration, because of his failure in math and reading, will erupt into some other unacceptable behaviour. The failures have to be dealt with.

(6) Task or behaviour analysis is the breaking down of a whole skill or behaviour into its component parts and recognizing the logical sequence that takes place in learning the parts. Parents are often impatient when they teach a child a skill and the child is just not meeting the parent's expectation. This usually leads to frustrations of both parent and child, and the emotionality does not help the child to learn or the parent to teach. The explanation for the non-learning may be: (a) the instructions are not clear, or (b) the information is made up of indigestible chunks, i.e., it's too much material for this young brain to process.

Task analysis helps you to break down a task or behaviour into digestible bits or chunks so they can be absorbed, and this leads to success, which becomes the basis for more success. For example, if you intend to teach your child how to swim, carry out a task analysis on the skill of swimming or consult a manual. Swimming includes such component parts as learning how to breathe in water, kicking, using your arms, and then putting all these parts together into the whole, which is the swimming movement.

(7) It's also helpful to recognize the three stages in the learning process. It helps you to be more patient if you understand the Learning-Hope Curve.

In the beginning of learning (A to B), there is little performance, and dissatisfaction and frustration prevail. Be patient or this A-to-B period can be a time of difficulty and dropout. With good instruction and practice, performance takes off and B to C is a period of satisfaction,

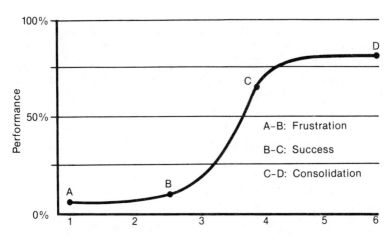

Figure 24. The Learning-Hope Curve

success, and elation. The Learning Curve is a Hope Curve and based on thousands of learning experiments, and it says: I know it's difficult and frustrating, but with time and practice I promise you that you will do better and better.

Other alternatives to hitting, yelling, nagging, and insult include the following. (8) Use behaviour management, its well-tested procedures, and its focus on reinforcing positive behaviours. (9) Examine your attitude toward your children. Are you just trying to catch bad behaviour or do you focus on and "catch" and reward the good behaviours? Some parents operate like prison guards, always on the lookout for trouble, which generally results in a self-fulfilling prophecy. (10) Establish a good family contract with clear limits, rules, privileges, responsibilities, and consequences. (11) Develop one-to-one relationships with your children where there is an ease and time for good communication, where bonding and binding take place, and where parents and children are partners and not protagonists. (12) Examine and re-examine your rating of your child's inappropriate behaviour. Your reaction to 10's are costly to your child, to your relationship with your child, and to your own feelings of inadequacy and self-esteem.

Finally, (13) run an *ABC Cost-Benefit Analysis* to determine the *cost* of your reaction, the *benefit* of your reaction, and your *alternatives* to this reaction. For example:

A: *The Cause.* Jamie forgot his homework at school gain.

B: *Your Behaviour.* You yell at him.

C: *The Consequence.* It widens the rift between you and Jamie. You feel guilty. He still forgets his homework.

193

The conclusion, obviously, is that there have been no benefits and the costs are great.

But there are alternatives to this fruitless chain of events. First, *identify* who owns the problem. It is Jamie's problem. Have you assumed his problem? Second, *listen* to him, in a one-to-one situation without being judge or jury. Try to establish a climate where he can share what is happening to him without fear of reprimand or loss of self-esteem, where he feels you are listening empathetically and that he will not be subjected to yelling, criticism, or preaching. The problem might be:

- I can never remember to bring my homework home.
- I don't understand the work at school and I can't do it. I'd rather be criticized for forgetting my homework than look like a dummy in front of all my friends.
- My friends never take a book home. I don't want to be different.
- I'm too busy with my paper route, my basketball practice, and looking after my house jobs – I don't have any time for my homework.
- I can't stand having you and Dad constantly looking over my shoulder when I do my homework.
- It's so noisy and busy in our house I can't concentrate.

By allowing Jamie to be open without any concern, the problem can surface and everyone's preoccupation is with solutions, not reprimand. *There are solutions.*

Your goal is to see that Jamie owns his problems, understands the consequences of his problems, and learns to develop strategies to solve them. By being able to share his problems and concerns, he learns that they take on some clarity. It really helps to bounce possible solutions off someone who listens, trusts, and who may be able to help him explore other alternatives.

In sum, your alternative behaviours include: (1) Let your child own his problems. (2) Establish a climate where you become the empathetic listener and where your child feels at ease, open, and accepting of your help.

As another example, let's look at Kim, who is fifteen years old and thirty-one pounds overweight. Her self-esteem is at an all-time low. She hates herself and has become a loner. She doesn't care about her clothes, her room, or her schoolwork. Kim's parents have encouraged her to go on a diet and have changed their own eating habits by cutting out ice cream, cakes, cookies, and all the carbohydrate goodies in the house. They sent her to a special camp and to different physicians and nutritionists. They have scolded, threatened, and yelled at her. Nothing worked!

A: The Cause. While Kim was at school, her mother decided to clean her room. In the back of Kim's cupboard, under a pile of clothes, Mom discovered a bag of chocolate bars, some caramel corn, and a banana peel! This caused Mom to react.

B: The Behaviour. When Kim came in from school her mother was in a rage and fired off with "You fat slob! You ingrate! Your room is fit for a pig and that describes you – a pig! There is a bag of chocolate bars and garbage in your room. Oh, how I wish you weren't mine!" Mother's patience had run out and she heaped insult upon invective upon more insult.

C: The Consequence. Kim sat on the floor and sobbed hysterically. "I just want to die. I hate you. You're a horrible mother!" The mother cried inside and hated herself for her impatient, cruel outburst. She felt horrible for destroying whatever was left of Kim's fragile self-esteem. She knew her yelling and her insults didn't help. They only served to shut off any communication. She loved this child so much she could feel her pain, and yet she seemed so helpless.

What are the mother's alternative behaviours here? What Kim needed was not a policewoman checking her room every day, nor a judge handing down sentences for her eating misdemeanours, nor abuse. She desperately needed someone she could talk to and share without fear of judgement.

There was now a wide rift between Kim and her mother and father. The only communication seemed to be reprimand and defensiveness and the central topic was always Kim's weight. It haunted her at home, at school, and everywhere. She felt that everyone looked at her with, "What a fat slob – you have no self-control!"

An alternative that I suggested to her parents and specifically to her mother was that they begin to park their focus on Kim's weight and Kim's eating habits. This focus was choking communication and any possible relationship. It was suggested that her mother try to arrange some one-to-one outings where they could just be together. At different times she suggested:

- "Kim, I have two tickets for the symphony Friday night. They are playing Chopin Nocturnes, your favourites."
- "Kim, I would like to redecorate the front hall. Would you come shopping with me and help me choose some new wallpaper and fixtures?"
- "I'm a little concerned about this lump in my breast. Would you come with me to my next doctor's appointment?"
- "Kim, I have a report to write and I would like to go to the cottage for the weekend. How about coming up with me?"

Kim said "no" to the first two but "yes" to the other two. Their relationship began to improve slowly, painfully, and hesitantly. In their one-to-one times together, Mother began to disclose herself to Kim, her teen-age dreams and the plans she once had, her romantic disappointments, and her great conquest – Dad. They laughed together, walked, and listened to each other, and their friendship grew. Mother's self-disclosures gave Kim licence to share herself, and she did.

It was difficult to avoid the subject of eating and weight, but it was parked. Eventually they became comfortable even in eating situations. Kim now felt that when her mother looked at her she did not look at her fat, but at what was inside. Kim felt accepted and loved and, one day, Kim was ready. "Mom, I am going to lose twenty-five pounds and I'm going to do it this time – there's no question about it. I'm going to succeed! I need your support. I have a good nutritional program, no crash diets. I've joined the physical fitness program at school and I wondered if you would like to join the "Y" with me and learn how to play badminton?"

Kim now owned the problem and made the decision. She recognized that the support and love of her parents would help her achieve her goal, but no one else could do it for her.

What were the alternative behaviours here? These included (a) getting off Kim's back and *parking* the preoccupation with Kim's weight, and (b) a one-to-one relationship where mother began to *see* Kim, to *listen* to her, and where they learned to *share* their tears and laughter and to build a loving bond.

If your genes didn't gift you with patience, it still can be acquired. This takes time, understanding, and practice of the strategies that can prevent or minimize the impatient behaviours affecting your enjoyment and fulfilment of being a parent and a person.

Summary: A Four-step Strategy for Patience

STEP 1: THE CAUSE

Examine the "why" of your child's behaviour that caused you to lose your patience. Was it intentional or accidental? Does it occur frequently? If you can understand and eliminate the *cause* of the behaviour you have eliminated the behaviour that upsets you.

STEP 2: CHECK YOUR RATING

Check the accuracy of your rating or evaluation of the seriousness of this "bad behaviour." Is it a 10 or is it a 3? Or is it somewhere in between? Your reaction depends on this evaluation. Check the factors that affect this evaluation and your patience level:

- the accuracy of your perception
- your present physical, mental, and emotional condition
- your values, motives, and expectations
- your understanding of child development
- your skills in dealing with the problems of development
- your past history in dealing with similar problems

These factors all affect your rating of your children's behaviour and misbehaviour. *Patience increases and your rating decreases.*

STEP 3: THE EMOTIONAL REACTION

Allow yourself to be angry. Let your kids know you're upset and why, but don't let yourself be *preoccupied* with your anger since it takes away from your ability to solve the problem and change behaviour. If you are carrying around too much pressure, use a *stress reduction* procedure: ventilation, positive self-statements, muscle relaxation, biofeedback, physical activity, music, a hobby, humour, or prayer.

STEP 4: YOUR PHYSICAL AND VERBAL REACTION

Check out your alternatives to hitting, yelling, and nagging. Patience develops when you:

1. Actively and empathetically listen to your child.
2. Can suggest and offer alternative methods of dealing with the problems of your children.
3. Have clear contracts, clear limits, and clear consequences.
4. Acknowledge and reinforce appropriate behaviour.
5. Understand how children learn – i.e., the Learning-Hope Curve.
6. Learn to teach by using a task analysis, i.e., breaking the learning into small chunks so that they can succeed.
7. Develop one-to-one relationships with your children so that you understand each other better, communicate better, and enjoy each other more.
8. Run an ABC Cost-Benefit Analysis to check the effectiveness of

your present behaviour and to explore alternative behaviours that may resolve the problem.

9. Set an example of appropriate behaviour. Don't just preach it – do it!

10. Get some distance from your children from time to time. Schedule a vacation without them. You'll appreciate them more and they will appreciate you.

TWELVE

Epilogue

We make a number of major decisions in our lifetime and many of these decisions can be reversed. You can buy a car, get tired of it, and trade it in; you can buy a house, which is a major investment decision, feel it's inadequate, and sell it; you can enter a career, become disenchanted or bored, and change it – there is no calamitous consequence to the reversal in your decision. Even marriage, which is one of the most critical decisions in your life, may not work out. And in today's society some 35-50 per cent reverse this decision and go their own ways, sometimes for good reasons and sometimes for lack of effort, commitment, or impulsiveness.

But the decision to have children is final and irreversible. You can't trade them in, sell them, abandon them, or wish them away. They are your property for at least eighteen years of their lives. Society and the laws are there to enforce ownership. The laws, however, are lax when it comes to the care of this property and so you can abuse, punish, neglect, and totally control your children's lives until they reach adulthood. It takes severe child abuse before laws will get involved. Society and the law do not require any test of competency for this major decision and responsibility.

Why do most of us make the decision to have children? As indicated in the first chapter herein, there are positive and negative motives for this decision. Some individuals have fatalistic motivations and believe that having children is the reason for their existence and to decide not to have them is a sin against God and country. Others want to ensure the continuation of their family name, and in a previous age many had children for such economic reasons as helping around the farm and the house. Some parents have children because they need to be needed, to keep their marriage together, for emotional stability, or to achieve the successes they didn't achieve.

Others decide to have children for more positive motives. They just love and enjoy kids and have developed some understanding of child development and some skills for parenting, or they may have so enjoyed

199

their childhood and their parents that they want to repeat the experience.

For some there was no decision – it was just an accident. As our research indicates, the motive to have a child is a reasonable prediction for the success in parenting: the more positive the motive, the more positive the outcome. Nevertheless, regardless of the motive it is a long-term, challenging, and difficult responsibility. As Virginia Satir suggests, "parents teach in the toughest school in the world – The School of Making People – and there are few schools to train you and there is no general agreement on the curriculum. There are no holidays, no vacations or pay raises. You are on duty or at least on call twenty-four hours a day, 365 days a year, for at least eighteen years for each child you have.... I regard this as the hardest, most complicated, anxiety-ridden, sweat-and-blood-producing job in the world. It requires the ultimate in patience, common sense, honour, tact, love, wisdom, awareness, and knowledge. At the same time it holds the possibility for the most rewarding, joyous experience of a lifetime." Unfortunately, it is not a joyous experience for perhaps 41 per cent who report that for them it is a frustrating and negative experience.

The decision to have children is easy, the biological act of conception is easy and pleasant, but the responsibilities that follow are not easy. Child-rearing is more complicated than flying a jetliner, operating a computer, or taking out someone's tonsils. We wouldn't dream of making a decision to fly a plane without years of training. When will we recognize that though parenting may begin with love and affection it is not sufficient? Some expertise is needed and this expertise is not instinctive. Inexperienced parenting is costly to the parent, to the child (who was not even party to your decision), and to society. There are millions of messed-up kids who become messed-up adults.

Most parents have abdicated their role as the first teacher and the central agent in a child's life to society, the school system, the church, the street, movies, television, welfare agencies, and professionals. The fathers have been traditionally the "supreme" abdicators – only 7 per cent have ever read a book on parenting. They judiciously avoid lectures and workshops, and for them "parent education" means "mother education." Millions of "how to fix it" books are bought and read by fathers on everything from "how to improve your lawn" to "how to replace your toilet bowl" but they don't buy or read a book on "how to raise your kids."

What is amazing is that we know the cost of poor parenting in terms of the emotional, learning, and behavioural disorders, delinquency, alcohol and drug addiction, and teen pregnancies and disease. Hundreds of studies relate parenting styles and parenting behaviour to children's behaviour. We have data on the sequential stages of emotional, intellectual, moral, and social personality development and on the type of environment that facilitates optimum growth at each stage. There are well-tested methods to help children become self-disciplined and motivated and to learn. Though no specific recipe exists for successful parenting, the information we have gives us good direction and eliminates much of the trial and error.

We have all this *technology* to teach and to prevent many of the problems of poor parenting but we have not translated the decision to have a child into a decision to learn how to care for and raise the child. By default it's a decision to have someone else be responsible for raising, teaching, and fixing. Professionals, such as a child's teacher, are overwhelmed with the responsibility of being the prime teacher and the fixer and many recognize that they can never be the central agent in a child's life. They can't even do a repair job without the parents' co-operation.

A child has the sacred right to parental love and parental expertise and even this is not enough. A child has the right to parents who are reasonably well-adjusted and stable and whose marriage is a growing, healthy, affectionate partnership.

As a professional, I have over the years assumed the role of repairman but without involved parents it's patchwork repair. I used to think that we were only dealing with small numbers of children because there are only a limited number of repair facilities. We are not; there are millions of kids and their parents who need help and the professionals are not curing or eliminating the problem. Government cannot legislate nor can schools educate away the ills. Statistics indicate the situation is getting worse, and if the trend continues the 41 per cent frustrated parents will become 51 and then 61 per cent. This book has been an attempt to share information and strategies for parenting that have been successful for the 22 per cent who found parenting fulfilling and enjoyable. The principles and strategies that were included are meant to give direction and encouragement to parents as individuals, as marriage partners, and in their central role in child-rearing. The understanding of motivation, self-concept, self-discipline, learning styles, contracts, the development of patience, the role of expectations: this breadth of understanding is as crucial for parents' growth as it is for the growth of children. Two hugs for survival are needed at all ages.

How did civilization survive for so long without parent education or parent training. Not very well! Today we are in a position to assess the successes, the failures, and the costs. And because society is more complex than it was a hundred years ago there are many more failures. Some children are resilient and grow up well in spite of their environment; many do not.

Some of the learnings for good parenting are new; most have been around and are only now being documented. It is not suggested that all the learning and training can come from courses or books. There are the 22 per cent of our parents in every community who have been successful and who should act as models. They are the real professionals who should be involved in parent training.

Finally, if parenting is so involved, so difficult, so consuming for so many years, and perhaps even potentially dangerous, why bother? Let me park my role as a psychologist and assume my favourite and most comfortable role – the father of Karen, Nancy, and Marilyn. They can best help me answer the question, why parenthood? I am not certain that there are words or language to describe adequately my feelings of love for them – or my gratefulness for our shared experiences and their love. They opened a deep reservoir of affection and caring. It was a love affair from the first moment I held and cuddled each of them at birth. I was overwhelmed with an awareness that I had been part of the creation of this new life, with a wonderment of what they would be like, with a realization of the awesome responsibility that came with this totally dependent being, and with a commitment that "I will take care of you." I was and am overwhelmed.

The growing years were wondrous and forever changing; they were years of joy and pain: the pain that comes from all-night vigils with fevers, coughs, croup, mumps, bruises, fears, bad dreams, and growing pains. These experiences tried and tested and seemed only to bond us closer.

What magic there is to the spontaneous "I love you, Daddy!" A walk down the street with that little, warm, trusting hand in yours; to the precious good-night ritual of the bedtime story, "now I lay me down to sleep..." a kiss, and a hug. Their hugs truly helped survival and growth. It has been a voyage of excitement, of exhilaration, of concern, of learning, of discovery, of some success and some failures – but never disenchantment. We helped *each other* grow; and it's a process that continues to the present. Though they are now adults, with their own careers and their own families, they are still my dearest, closest, and most trusted friends.

There is something deeply innate about the need for self-fulfilment. It's a question and a search that is pervasive and elusive. Few really taste of it in their work or in their relationships. Some, in their quest, turn to "doing good" in the community through charity, church, youth or hospital committees, and the like; the others turn to self-indulgence. Both turns may be detours and empty. The road to self-fulfilment is often missed because it's so close to us – it's right at home. There are no headlines, no public notice or public acclaim to the parenting role. If it is assumed with commitment, preparation, involvement, affection, and faith, it leads to great "peak" experience.

Being part of creation and the growth of a child, the architect of the child's environment, the provider of the first basic needs, the teacher, playmate, model, and friend is the *ultimate* in self-fulfilment. This is the "magic formula," and though only 22 per cent may have found it, it's there, it's worthwhile, and the dividends are beyond measure.

Bibliography

Argyle, Michael. *The Psychology of Interpersonal Behavior*. London: Penguin Books, 1974.

Baumrind, Diana. *The Development of Instrumental Competence Through Socialization*. In Ann Peck (ed.), Minnesota Symposia on Child Psychology (Vol. 7). Minneapolis: University of Minnesota Press, 1973.

Becker, W. "The Consequences of Different Kinds of Parental Discipline," in M. Hoffman (ed.), *Review of Child Developmental Research*, Vol. 1 (New York: Russel Sage, 1964), 169-208.

Bigner, J. *Parent-Child Relations*. New York: Macmillan Publishing Company, 1979.

Bing, E. "Effect of Child Rearing Practices on the Development of Differential Cognitive Abilities," *Child Development* , 34 (1963), 631-648.

Blanchard, R., and H. Biller. "Father Availability and Academic Performance among 3rd Grade Boys," *Developmental Psychology*, 4 (1971), 301-305.

Bowlby, John. "The Nature of the Child's Tie to His Mother," *International Journal of Psychoanalysis*, 39 (1958), 35.

Briggs, Dorothy C. *Your Child's Self-Esteem*. New York: Doubleday Books, 1970.

Brown, A. *The Normal Child: Its Care and Feeding*. New York: Century Company, 1923.

Byrne, D. *An Introduction to Personality*. Englewood Cliffs, New Jersey: Prentice Hall, 1974.

Carlsmith, J.M., and E. Aronson, "Some Hedonic Consequences of the Confirmation and Disconfirmation of Expectancies," *Journal of Abnormal and Social Psychology*, 66 (1963), 151-156.

Celdic Report. *One Million Children - The Celdic Report*. Toronto: Leonard Crawford Publisher, 1970.

Chapman, A.H. *Management of Emotional Problems of Children and Adolescents*. Philadelphia: Lippincott, 1965.

Chess, Stella, Alexander Thomas, and Herbert G. Birch. *Your Child is a Person*. New York: Penguin Books, 1976.

Coopersmith, Stanley. *The Antecedents of Self-Esteem*. San Francisco: W.H. Freeman, 1967.

Dreikurs, Rudolph. *Children: The Challenge*. Des Moines: Meredith Press, 1964.

Elkind, David. *The Child and Society*. New York: Oxford University Press, 1979.

Erikson, Erik H. *Childhood and Society* (2nd ed.). New York: Norton, 1963.

Fromm, Erich. *The Art of Loving*. New York: Harper & Row, 1956.

Ginott, Haim G. *Between Parent and Child*. New York: Avon Books, 1965.

Ginott, Haim G. *Between Parent and Teenager*. New York: Avon Books, 1971.

Gordon, Thomas. *P.E.T. Parent Effectiveness Training*. New York: New American Library, 1975.

Harlow, Harry F. "The Nature of Love," *American Psychologist*, 13 (1958).

Harlow, Harry F., and R.P. Zimmerman. "Affectional Responses in the Infant Monkey," *Science*, 130 (1959), 421.

Hess, R., and V. Shipman. "Early Experience and Socialization of Cognitive Modes in Children," *Child Development*, 36 (1965), 869.

Hetherington, F. "Effects of Father Absence on Personality Development in Adolescent Daughters," *Developmental Psychology*, 7 (1972), 313-326.

Jersild, A.T. "Emotional Development," in L. Carmichael (ed.), *Manual of*

Child Psychology (New York: Wiley, 1946).

Jourard, S. "Identification, Parent Cathexis Self-esteem," *Journal of Consulting Psychology,* 21 (1957), 375-380.

Jourard, Sidney M. *The Transparent Self.* New York: D. Van Nostrand, 1964.

Jourard, Sidney M. *Disclosing Man to Himself.* New York: D. Van Nostrand, 1968.

Kagan, J., and H. Moss. *Birth to Maturity.* New York: Wiley, 1962.

Killory, J.F. "In Defence of Corporal Punishment," *Psychological Reports,* 35 (1974), 575-581.

Klein, Carole. *How it Feels to be a Child.* New York: Harper & Row, 1975.

Kohlberg, Lawrence. "The Development of Children's Orientations Toward a Moral Order: Sequence in the Development of Moral Thought," *Vita Humana,* 6 (1963).

Lanza, F.R. "An Investigation of Various Antecedents of Self-esteem as Related to Race and Sex." *Dissertation Abstracts International,* 31 (1970), 1077.

Lindsley, Ogden. *In Helping Parents Help Their Children.* Edited by E. Arnold. New York: Brunner Mazel Publishers, 1978.

Mandel, Harvey P., and Sander I. Marcus. "Early Infantile Autism: A Pre Ego Psychopathology and Case Report," *Psychotherapy: Theory, Research and Practice,* 8, 2 (1971).

Minuchin, S. *Families and Family Therapy.* Cambridge, Mass.: Harvard University Press, 1974.

Mussinger, H. *Fundamentals of Child Development.* New York: Holt, Rinehart & Winston, 1975.

Patterson, G.R. *Families' Application of Social Learning to Family Life.* Champaign, Illinois: Research Press, 1979.

Piaget, Jean. *The Moral Judgement of the Child.* New York: Harcourt Brace, 1932.

Piaget, Jean. *The Psychology of Intelligence.* London: Rutledge and Kegan, 1950.

Piaget, Jean, and Borkel Inhelder. *The Psychology of the Child.* New York: Basic Books, 1969.

Prescott, James W. "Alienation of Affection," *Psychology Today* (December, 1979).

Radke, M.J. *Relation of Parental Authority to Children's Behavior and Attitudes.* Minneapolis: University of Minnesota, Institute of Child Welfare Monograph 22, 1946.

Ribble, Margaret. "Infantile Experiences in Relation to Personality Development," in J. McV. Hunt (ed.), *Personality and Behavior Disorders* (New York: Ronald Press, 1944).

Rosenthal, Robert. "Self-fulfilling Prophecy," in *Readings in Developmental Psychology Today* (Del Mar, California: CRM Books, 1968).

Rosenthal, Robert, and Lenore Jacobson. *Pygmalion in the Classroom.* New York: Holt, Rinehart & Winston, 1968.

Rousseau, Jean Jacques. *The First and Second Discourses.* Edited and translated by R. Masters. New York: St. Martin Press, 1964.

Satir, Virginia. *Cojoint Family Therapy.* Palo Alto: Science & Behavior Books, 1964.

Sears, R.R. "Relation of Early Socialization Experiences to Self Concepts and Gender Role in Middle Childhood," *Child Development,* 40 (1970), 267-289.

Sears, R.R., E. Maccoby, and H. Levin. *Patterns of Child Rearing.* Evanston, Illinois: Row Peterson, 1957.

Spitz, R. "Hospitalism," in O. Fenichel (ed.), *The Psychoanalytic Study of the Child,* Vol. 1 (New York: International University Press, 1945).

Spock, Benjamin. *Baby and Child Care.* New York: Pocket Books, 1976.

Storr, Anthony. "An International and Interdisciplinary Study," in S.N. Katz (ed.), *Family Violence* (Toronto: Butterworth, 1977).

Storr, Catherine. "Freud and the Concept of Parental Guilt," in Jonathan Miller (ed.), *Freud: The Man, His World, His Influence* (Boston: Little Brown, 1972), 98.

Thomas, Alexander, and Stella Chess. *Temperament and Development*. New York: Brunner Mazel, 1977.

Wood, John. *How Do You Feel. A Guide to Your Emotions*. Englewood Cliffs, New Jersey: Prentice Hall, 1974.